15-Minute Ketogenic Diet Meals

Quick & Easy 15-Minute Ketogenic Meals Using Simple Ingredients That Burns Fat 4x Faster

Ted Duncan

Table of Contents

Introduction v

Chapter 1   Quick Ketogenic Breakfasts 8

Chapter 2   Quick Ketogenic Lunches 52

Chapter 3   Quick Ketogenic Dinners 92

Chapter 4   Quick Ketogenic Snacks 128

Conclusion 164

© Copyright 2018 by Ted Duncan - All rights reserved.

The follow eBook is reproduced below with the goal of providing information that is as accurate and reliable as possible. Regardless, purchasing this eBook can be seen as consent to the fact that both the publisher and the author of this book are in no way experts on the topics discussed within and that any recommendations or suggestions that are made herein are for entertainment purposes only. Professionals should be consulted as needed prior to undertaking any of the action endorsed herein.

This declaration is deemed fair and valid by both the American Bar Association and the Committee of Publishers Association and is legally binding throughout the United States.

Furthermore, the transmission, duplication or reproduction of any of the following work including specific information will be considered an illegal act irrespective of if it is done electronically or in print. This extends to creating a secondary or tertiary copy of the work or a recorded copy and is only allowed with express written consent from the Publisher. All additional right reserved.

The information in the following pages is broadly considered to be a truthful and accurate account of facts and as such any inattention, use or misuse of the information in question by the reader will render any resulting actions solely under their purview. There are no scenarios in which the publisher or the original author of this work can be in any fashion deemed liable for any hardship or damages that may befall them after undertaking information described herein.

Additionally, the information in the following pages is intended only for informational purposes and should thus be thought of as universal. As befitting its nature, it is presented without assurance regarding its prolonged validity or interim quality. Trademarks that are mentioned are done without written consent and can in no way be considered an endorsement from the trademark holder.

Introduction

I want to thank you and congratulate you for downloading 15-Minute Ketogenic Diet Meals. Taking control of your health and wellbeing can be a daunting task, but choosing this book will help you make these adjustments without feeling like you have to spend your life in the kitchen. This book will also show you that it also does not mean you have to give up some of your favorite foods and "treats!" With a few swaps in the ingredient list, hopefully, you will not be able to tell much of difference and continue to enjoy eating. But this time you can enjoy eating and being healthier.

The ketogenic lifestyle is a dietary choice that focuses on low to carbohydrates, acceptable amounts of protein and high fat. This approach encourages the body to use fat as energy, not carbohydrates. It accomplishes this internal reorganization by the metabolism that creates ketone bodies. These ketone bodies that are created are actually three compounds that occur when fat is burned. Carbohydrates have been linked to various negative health results, including poor insulin regulation that can result in type 2 diabetes. Taking control of your bodies energy and health can help you keep those various diseases at bay and shed weight in the meantime.

This book contains a variety of recipes that follow these dietary guidelines in 15 minutes or less. Occasionally a recipe may call for freeze time, but for the most part, these recipes you are about to explore are started and finished in 15 minutes or less. This means you now have an arsenal of recipes for whatever your taste buds desire that help you burn fat, lose weight, and feel better. Have fun trying new recipes and ingredients, your body will thank you!

Thanks again for downloading this book, I hope you enjoy it!

If you enjoy such content, click below to subscribe where we will send out self-improvement, non-fiction books, tips & information for you to read for FREE!

Do leave a good review as well if you found the content useful!

Click here ->http://eepurl.com/c5bzdX

Chapter 1
Quick Ketogenic Breakfasts

Breakfast Sandwich

This recipe makes 1 sandwich and requires about 10 minutes for cooking.

The serving size is 1 sandwich. It contains:

- *603 Calories*
- *54 g fat*
- *7 g total, 4 g net carbohydrates*
- *3 g fiber*
- *22 g protein*

What's in It

2	Sausage Patties
1 Tbsp	Cream cheese
2 Tbsp	Cheddar, sharp
½ tsp	Siracha
1	Egg
To taste	Salt
¼	Avocado, medium, sliced

How's it Made

1. Cook sausage patties according to directions on their packaging.

2. Microwave the cream cheese and cheddar until melted, about 30 seconds.
3. Stir in Siracha into the cheese mixture and set aside.
4. In a small bowl whisk the egg and salt, if using, until combined. Cook the eggs in a medium-hot skillet until fully cooked, about 4 minutes.
5. Remove the egg from the skillet and place on a plate. Top the egg with the cheese sauce, avocado and sausage. Fold over the top of the egg to make the sandwich and enjoy!

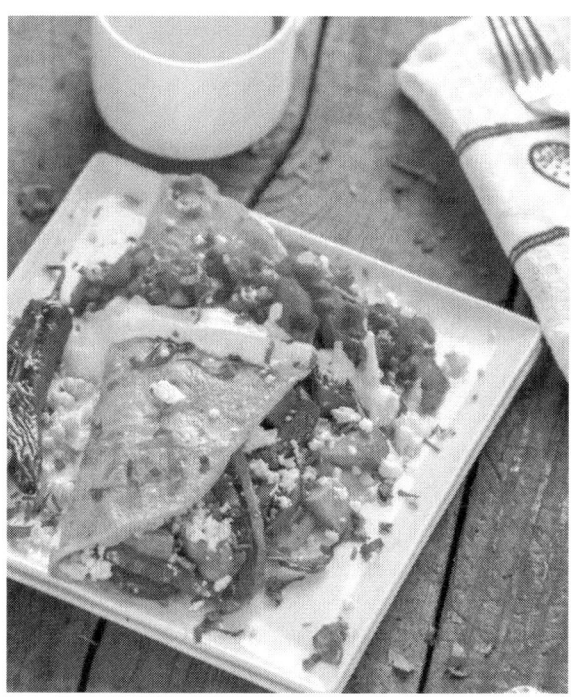

Omelet in a Mug

This recipe makes 1 omelet and requires about 2 minutes for cooking.

The serving size is 1 omelet. It contains:

- *284 Calories*
- *24 g fat*
- *4 g total, 3 g net carbohydrates*
- *1 g fiber*
- *15 g protein*

What's in It

As needed	Olive oil
2 or 3	Eggs
1 Tbsp	Meat, diced, such as ham
1 Tbsp	Salsa
1 Tbsp	Cheddar, sharp, shredded
To taste	Salt and pepper

How's it Made

1. In a large mug, rub the sides and bottom with olive oil.
2. Whisk the eggs inside the mug.
3. Whisk in the remaining ingredients until combined.
4. Place the mug in the microwave and cook on high for 1 minute.

5. Remove the mug and stir, breaking up large lumps of eggs.
6. Place the mug back into the microwave and cook on high for about 45 more seconds.
7. Sprinkle cheese and more salt and pepper on top, if desired.

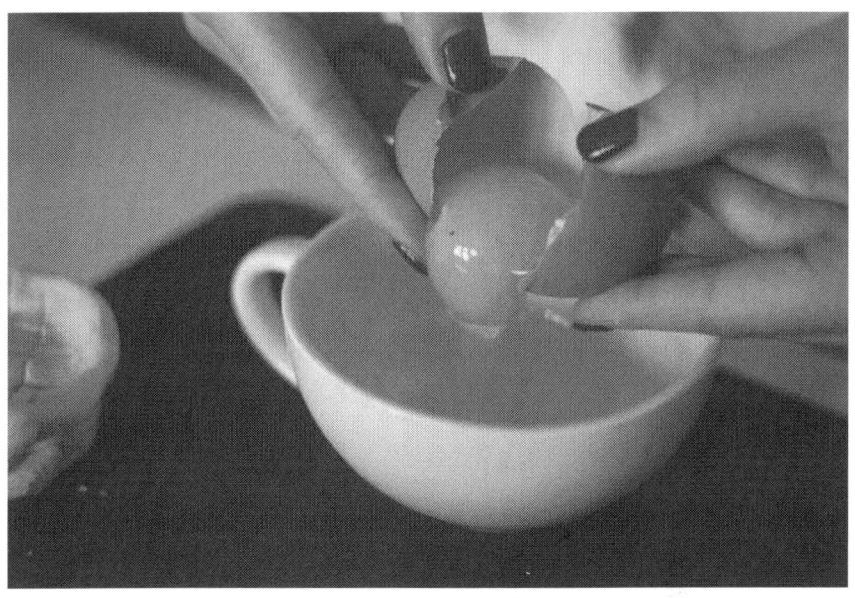

Egg and vegetable scramble

This recipe makes 1 scramble and requires about 2 minutes for cooking.

The serving size is 1 sandwich. It contains:

- *251 Calories*
- *20 g fat*
- *2 g total, 1.5 g net carbohydrates*
- *.5 g fiber*
- *17 g protein*

What's in It

As needed	Olive oil
3 or 4	Eggs
1 Cup	Spinach, fresh, raw
½ Cup	Vegetables, mixed, frozen
To taste	Salt and pepper

How's it Made

1. In a skillet over medium heat, heat up oil.
2. Add the frozen vegetables and cook for a few minutes to defrost and cook through.
3. Stir in eggs and add salt and pepper, if using.
4. Mix in the spinach and stir until wilted.
5. Remove from the skillet and tops with fresh spinach, if desired.

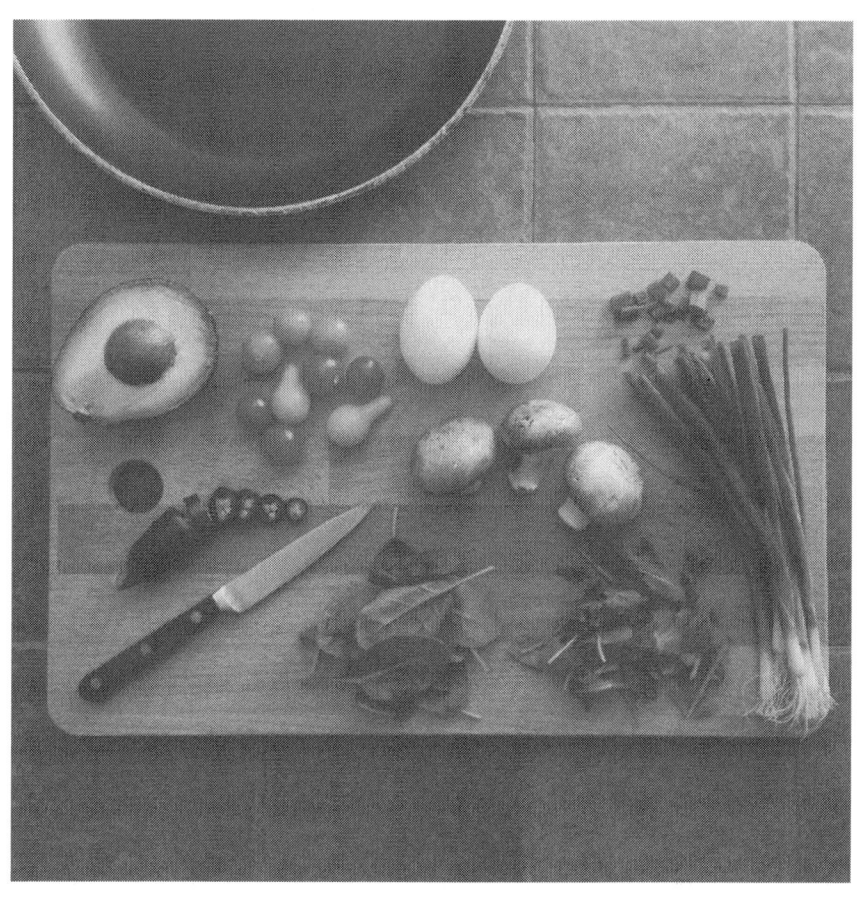

Breakfast Muffin

This recipe makes 1 muffin and requires about 2 minutes for cooking.

The serving size is 1 muffin. It contains:

- *113 Calories*
- *6 g fat*
- *5 g total, 2 g net carbohydrates*
- *3 g fiber*
- *7 g protein*

What's in It

As needed	Olive oil
1	Eggs
2 tsp	Coconut flour
Pinch	Baking soda
To taste	Salt

How's it Made

1. In a muffin tin or ramekin, grease with olive oil.
2. In a small bowl, whisk the remaining ingredients together until smooth and pour into the tin or ramekin.
3. Microwave on high for 1 minute or cook in a preheated oven at 400 degrees Fahrenheit for 12 minutes.

4. Remove from the tin and let cool. Cut in half to serve.

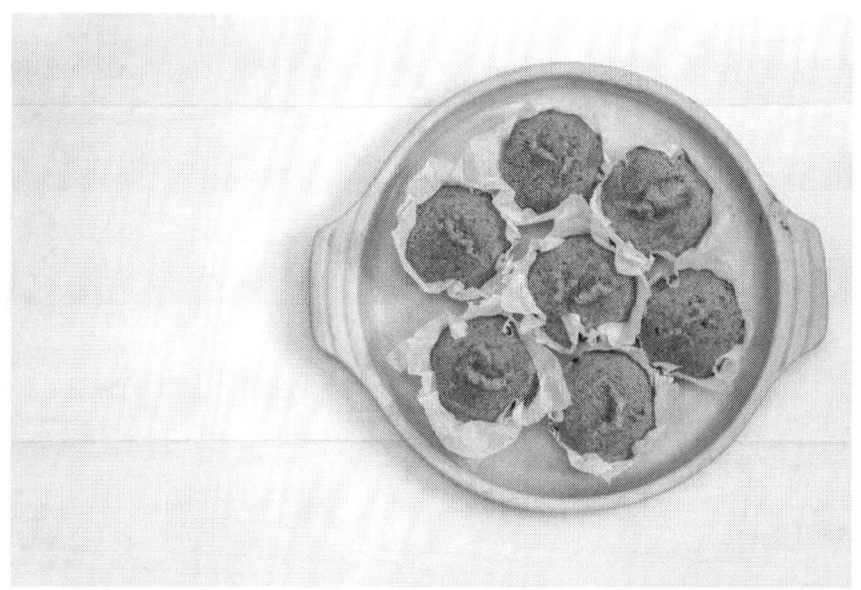

Crustless Spinach Quiche

This recipe makes 4 slices and requires about 15 minutes for cooking.

The serving size is 1 slice. It contains:

- *306 Calories*
- *18 g fat*
- *3 g total, 2.5 g net carbohydrates*
- *.5 g fiber*
- *32 g protein*

What's in It

1 Tbsp	Olive oil
2 Cups	Spinach, fresh, raw
8	Eggs
3 Cups	Cheddar, shredded
¼ tsp	Salt
¼ tsp	Pepper

How's it Made

1. Grease a small pan or muffin tins with the oil. Preheat the oven to 350 degrees Fahrenheit.
2. In a skillet over medium heat, warm about ½ tablespoon of oil and add the spinach, stirring until it is wilted and most of the water released is evaporated. Remove from the heat to cool.

3. In a small bowl, whisk the eggs, cheese, and seasoning until combined. Stir in the wilted and cooled spinach.
4. Pour the egg mixture into the greased pan or tins and bake in the oven for about 15 minutes. Baking in muffin tins or ramekins will be faster than in a pie or casserole dish.

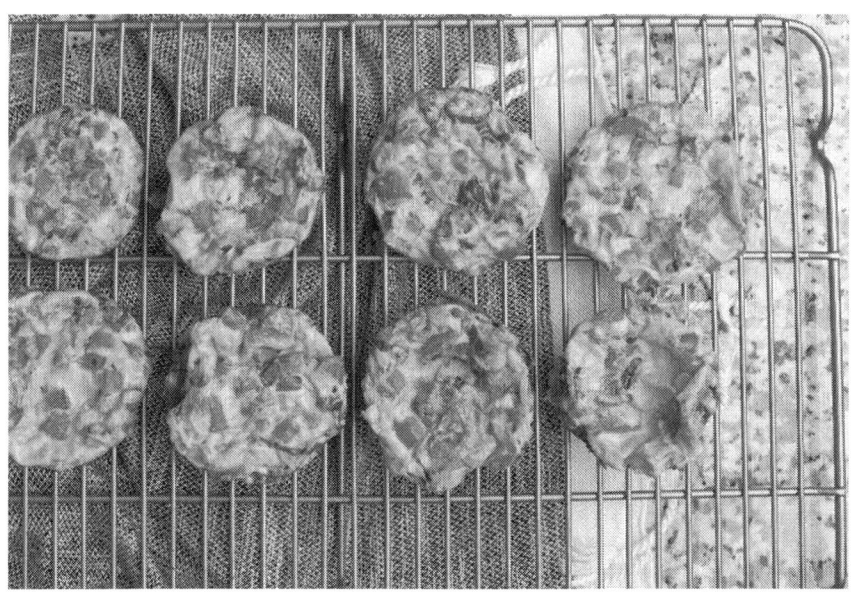

Avocado Breakfast Burger

This recipe makes 1 burger and requires about 15 minutes for cooking.

The serving size is 1 burger. It contains:

- *753 Calories*
- *65 g fat*
- *24 g total, 10 g net carbohydrates*
- *14 g fiber*
- *24 g protein*

What's in It

2 slices	Bacon
1	Egg
1	Avocado
1 Tbsp	Paleo Mayonnaise
1 leaf	Lettuce
1 slice	Tomato
1 slice	Red onion
To taste	Salt and pepper
As desired	Sesame seeds

How's it Made

1. Cook the bacon until crisp in a skillet over medium high heat. Remove from bacon from the pan and set aside.

2. In the same skillet, add the egg, cooking until the whites are cooked through but yolks are still loose.
3. Halve the avocado width-wise and remove the pit. Using a spoon, gently scoop the avocado from the skin.
4. Fill the avocado pit hole with mayonnaise.
5. On the bottom avocado layer add a layer of lettuce, a slice of tomato, a slice of onion, bacon and the fried egg.
6. Place the second half of the avocado on top and sprinkle with sesame seeds, if desired.

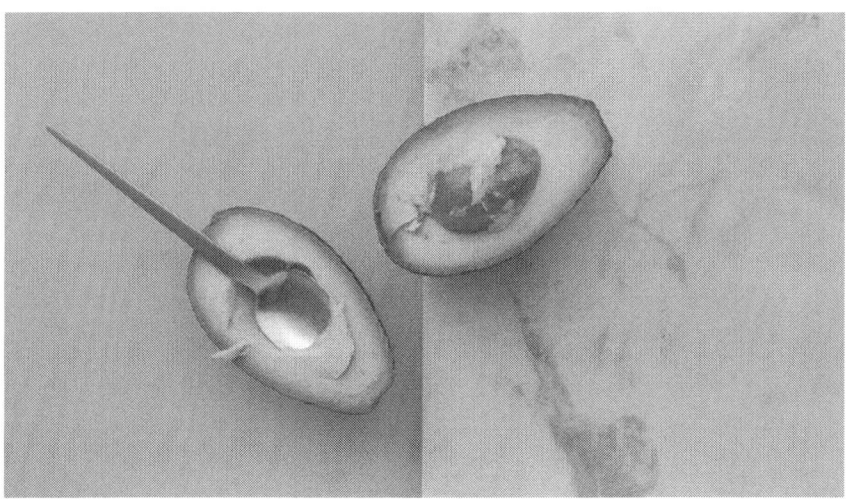

BLT Breakfast Salad

This recipe makes 2 servings and requires about 15 minutes for cooking.

The serving size is 1/2 salad. It contains:

- *292 Calories*
- *18 g fat*
- *18 g total, 11 g net carbohydrates*
- *7 g fiber*
- *18 g protein*

What's in It

3 Cups	Kale, shredded
1 tsp	Red wine vinegar
2 tsp	Olive oil
2	Eggs, cooked,
4 Slices	Bacon, cooked, chopped
2 Ozs	Avocado, sliced
10	Grape tomatoes, halved
To taste	Salt and pepper

How's it Made

1. Cook the bacon until crisp in a skillet over medium high heat. Remove the bacon from the pan and set aside.
2. Cook the egg in the skillet over medium high heat. Remove the egg from the pan and set aside.

3. In a bowl, mix by hand the kale, oil, vinegar and salt, if using. Mix until kale is tender. Place the salad mixture in two bowls.
4. Chop the bacon and place on top of the salads. Add the tomatoes, eggs and avocados to each salad. Sprinkle with pepper and mores salt, if desired.

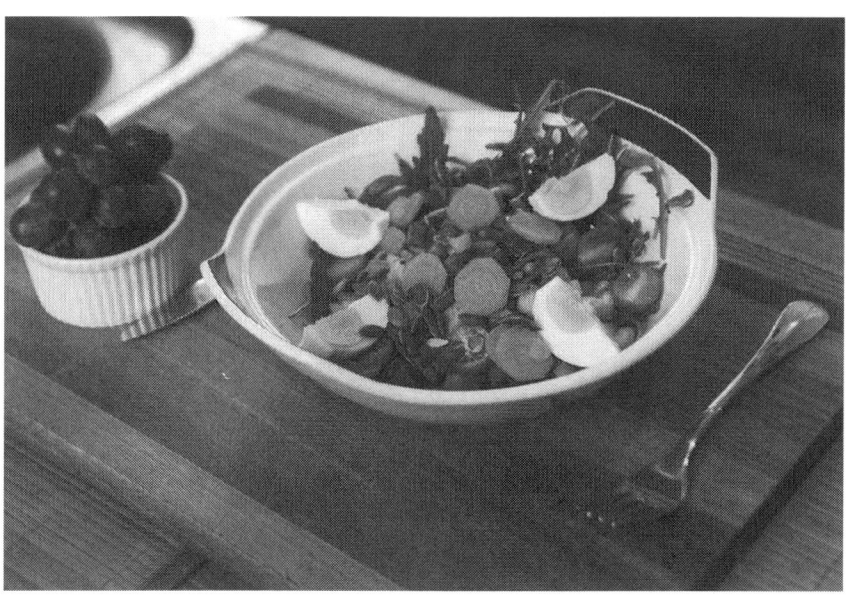

Hollandaise Egg Bake

This recipe makes 4 servings and requires about 15 minutes for cooking.

The serving size is 1 ramekin. It contains:

- *1271 Calories*
- *93 g fat*
- *13 g total, 12 g net carbohydrates*
- *1 g fiber*
- *94 g protein*

What's in It

2	Egg yolks
¼ C	Butter, melted
2 tsp	Lemon juice
¼ tsp	Salt
¼ tsp	Paprika
4 Ozs	Bacon, chopped
1 C	Mixed greens
8	Eggs

How's it Made

1. Prepare the hollandaise sauce: In a blender, combine the egg yolks, juice, paprika and salt until combined. While still blending, slowly add in the melted butter. Mix for about 30 seconds. Set aside.
2. Preheat the oven to 400 degrees Fahrenheit.

3. Cook the bacon in a skillet over medium heat until almost cooked through.
4. Stir in the greens and mix until wilted.
5. Portion out the greens and bacon into four ramekins or oven-safe dishes. Add one egg on top to each ramekin.
6. Bake each ramekin for about 10 minutes or until the whites are hard and the yolk is still slightly loose.
7. Top with hollandaise sauce.

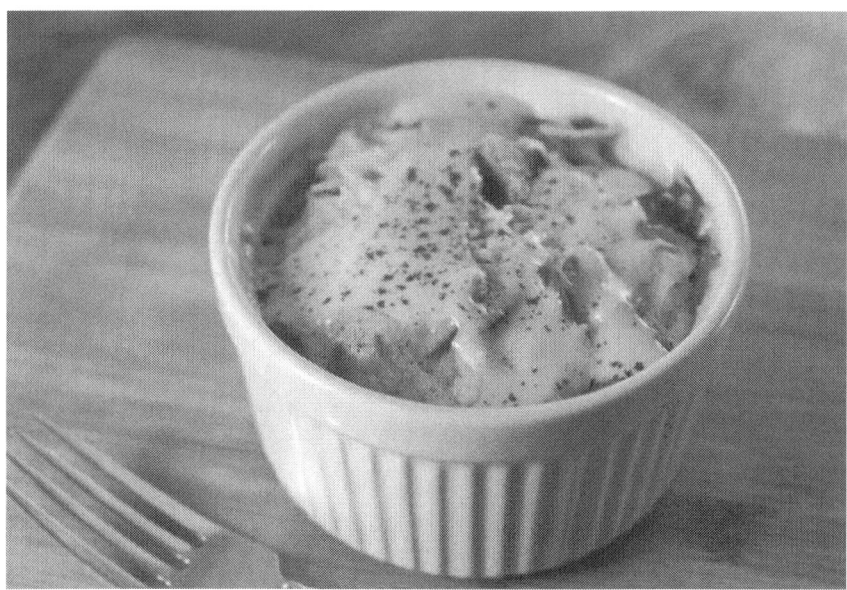

Egg and Avocado wrapped in Prosciutto

This recipe makes 2 servings and requires about 12 minutes for cooking.

The serving size is 1 avocado. It contains:

- *963 Calories*
- *72 g fat*
- *22 g total, 8 g net carbohydrates*
- *14 g fiber*
- *63 g protein*

What's in It

2	Eggs
2	Avocados
6 Slices	Prosciutto
2 Tbsp	Olive oil
To taste	Salt and pepper

How's it Made

1. Poach the eggs and set aside.
2. Flatten the prosciutto with a knife on a cutting board.
3. Halve lengthwise the avocado and remove the pit. Use a spoon to remove the avocado from the skin. Scoop out the inside of the avocado so the hole is the same size as a poached egg.

Place one egg in one avocado piece. Place the other piece of avocado on top.
4. Gently wrap the avocado and egg with prosciutto. Place two strips around it horizontally and one strip around it vertically. Repeat for the other avocado and egg.
5. In a skillet over medium-high heat, heat the oil and place the avocadoes in the pan, loose ends of the prosciutto facing down. Fry for about 10 minutes, turning often.
6. Remove from heat and sprinkle with salt and pepper before serving.

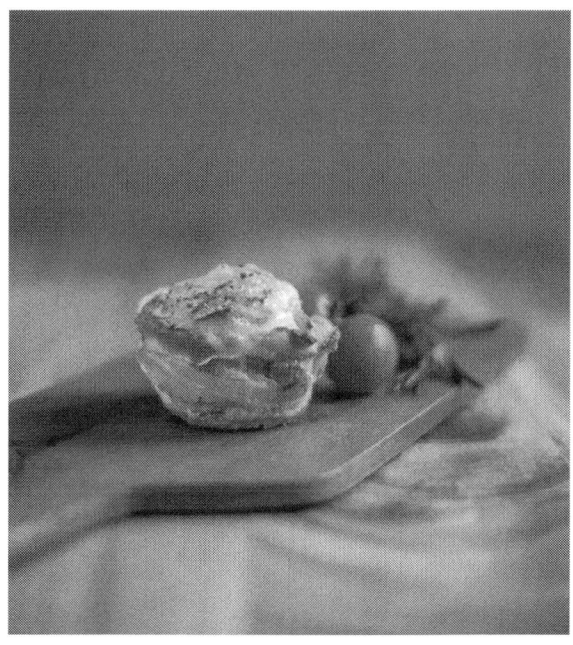

Cauli-fritters

This recipe makes 6 fritters and requires about 15 minutes for cooking.

The serving size is 1 fritter. It contains:

- *99 Calories*
- *7 g fat*
- *6 g total, 5 g net carbohydrates*
- *1 g fiber*
- *5 g protein*

What's in It

4 C	Cauliflower, riced
2	Eggs
2/3 C	Almond flour
1 Tbsp	Nutritional yeast
½ tsp	Turmeric
½ tsp	Salt
¼ tsp	Pepper
2 Tbsp	Butter

How's it Made

1. In a large bowl, mix all the ingredients except the butter until combined. Mold into 6 uniform patties.

2. In a skillet over medium heat, melt the butter. When melted, add each patty and cook on each side, about 4 minutes each.

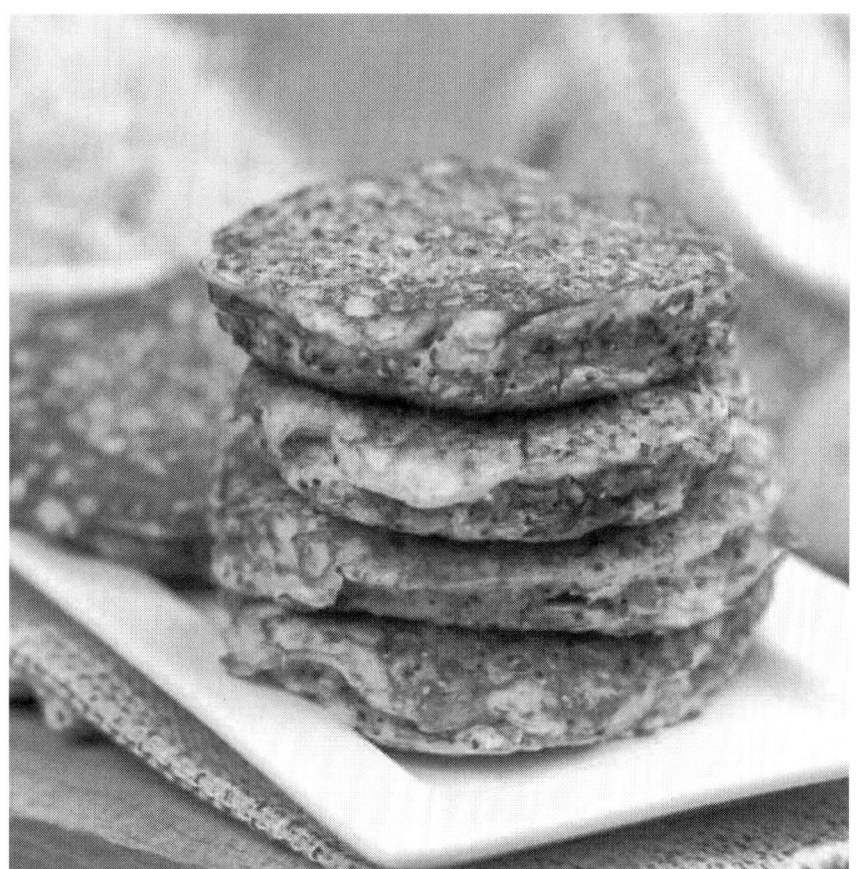

Zucc-fritters

This recipe makes 6 fritters and requires about 15 minutes for cooking.

The serving size is 1 fritter. It contains:

- *96 Calories*
- *7 g fat*
- *5 g total, 3 g net carbohydrates*
- *2 g fiber*
- *4 g protein*

What's in It

2 C	Broccoli florets, riced
1 C	Zucchini, grated, liquid removed
1/3 C	Scallion, chopped
2	Eggs, beaten
2 Tbsp	Basil, fresh, chopped
2/3 C	Almond flour
1 Tbsp	Nutritional yeast
½ tsp	Salt
2 Tbsp	Butter

How's it Made

1. In a large bowl, mix all the ingredients except the butter until combined. Mold into 6 uniform patties.

2. In a skillet over medium heat, melt the butter. When melted, add each patty and cook on each side, about 4 minutes each.

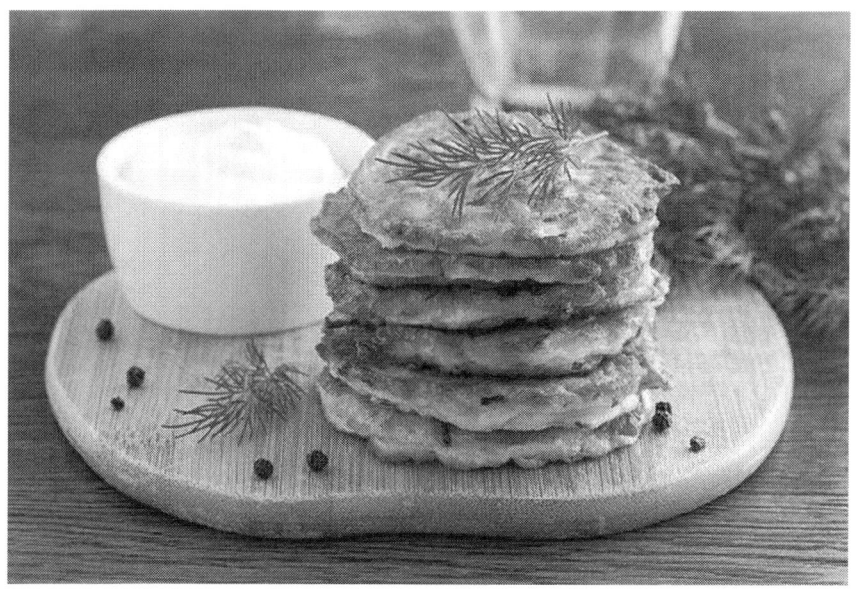

Brussels and Bacon Hash

This recipe makes 3 servings and requires about 12 minutes for cooking.

The serving size is 1/3 skillet. It contains:

- *220 Calories*
- *13 g fat*
- *12 g total, 8 g net carbohydrates*
- *4 g fiber*
- *17 g protein*

What's in It

12 Ozs	Brussels sprouts, sliced
2 Ozs	Bacon
2 Cloves	Garlic, minced
2	Shallots, minced
1 ½ Tbsp	Apple cider vinegar
3	Eggs
To taste	Salt and pepper

How's it Made

1. Over medium heat, cook the bacon in a skillet. Remove from heat.
2. In the same skillet, sauté the garlic and shallots for 30 seconds. Add the sliced Brussels sprouts and vinegar and stir to combine. Cook for 5 minutes, stirring often.

3. Add the bacon back to the skillet and continue to stir for another 3 minutes.
4. Create a hole in the middle of the skillet and add the eggs, cooking until they are cooked through.

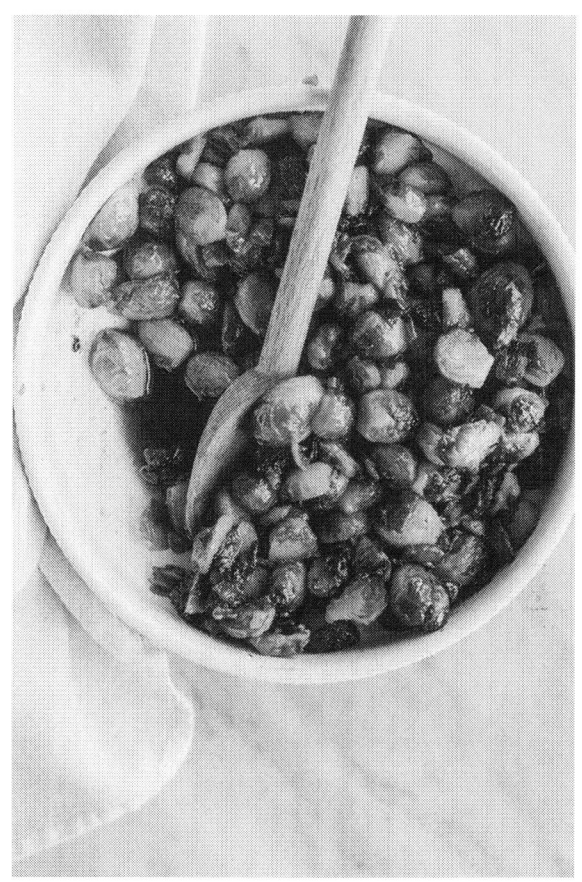

Coconut Porridge

This recipe makes 1 serving and requires about 7 minutes for cooking.

The serving size is 1 bowl. It contains:

- *453 Calories*
- *39 g fat*
- *14 g total, 5 g net carbohydrates*
- *9 g fiber*
- *13 g protein*

What's in It

2 Tbsp	Coconut flour
2 Tbsp	Flax meal
¾ C	Water
1	Egg
2 tsp	Butter
1 Tbsp	Heavy cream
1 Tbsp	Sugar or other sweetener
To taste	Salt
As desired	Fruit, nuts, granola, etc.

How's it Made

1. In a large pot, mix flour, meal, water and a pinch of salt over medium heat. When it simmers, lower the heat to medium-low and cook until it thickens, whisking constantly.

2. Remove the pot from the heat and whisk in the egg slowly. Put the pot back on the heat and keep whisking.
3. Remove the pot from the heat and whisk for 30 seconds. Add the butter, cream and sugar. Top with desired toppings.

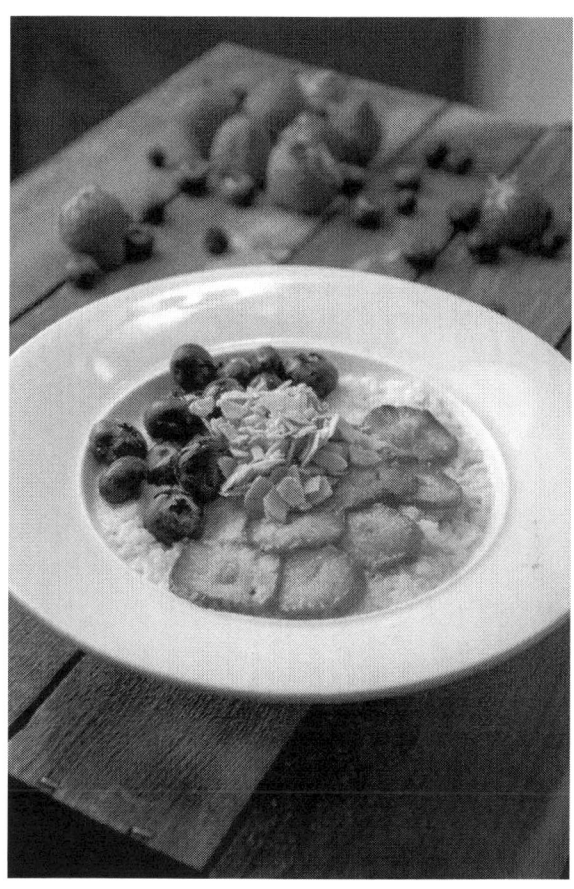

Dairy-Free Latte

This recipe makes 1 serving and requires about 3 minutes for cooking.

The serving size is 1 serving. It contains:

- *368 Calories*
- *36 g fat*
- *2 g total, 1 g net carbohydrates*
- *0 g fiber*
- *11 g protein*

What's in It

2	Eggs
2 Tbsp	Coconut oil
1 ½ C	Water, boiling
Dash	Vanilla exract
1 tsp	Pumpkin Pie spice

How's it Made

1. In a blender, mix all the ingredients and blend until creamy and smooth.

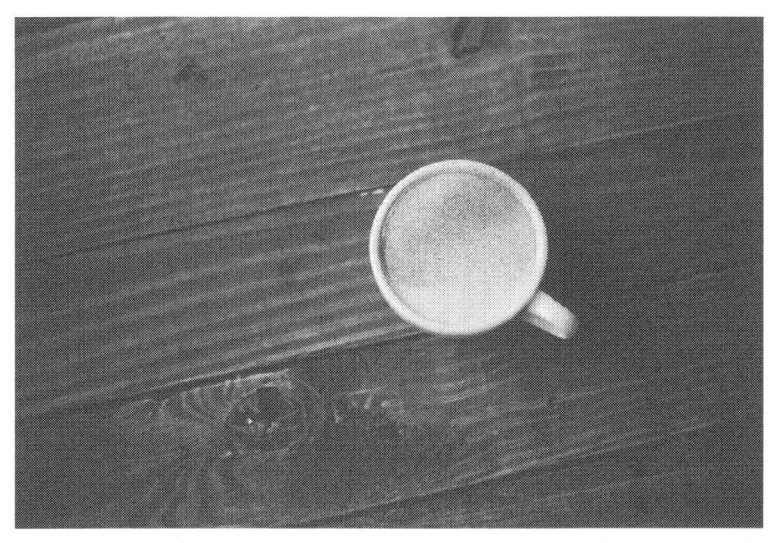

Salmon Scrambled Eggs

This recipe makes 1 serving and requires about 5 minutes for cooking.

The serving size is 1 plate. It contains:

- *738 Calories*
- *70 g fat*
- *15 g total, 14.5 g net carbohydrates*
- *.5 g fiber*
- *45 g protein*

What's in It

2	Eggs
2 Tbsp	Butter
4 tbsp	Whipping cream, heavy
1 Tbsp	Chives, fresh, chopped
2 Ozs.	Salmon, cured
To taste	Salt and pepper

How's it Made

1. In a small bowl, whisk the eggs.
2. In a skillet, melt the butter over medium heat. Add the whisked eggs and cream and stir constantly until cooked but creamy.
3. Transfer eggs to a plate and top with salmon, chives, and salt and pepper to taste.

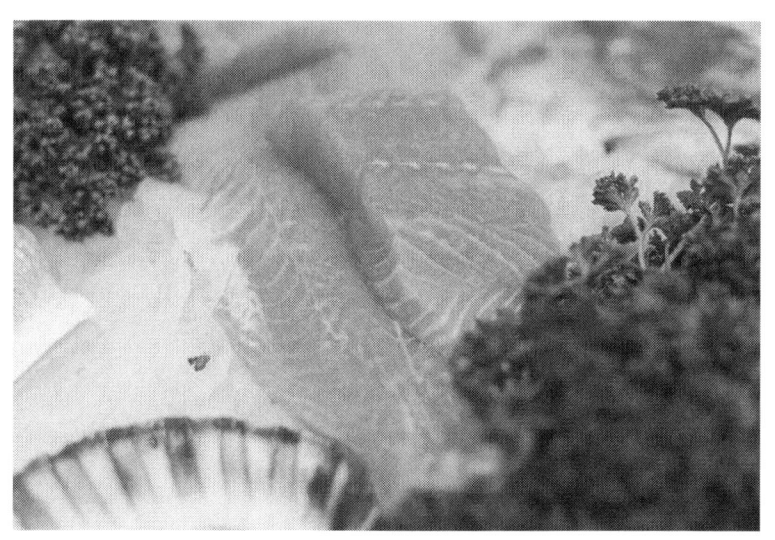

Tapas for Breakfast

This recipe makes 3 servings and requires about 5 minutes for cooking.

The serving size is 1/3 plate. It contains:

- *749 Calories*
- *58 g fat*
- *22 g total, 15 g net carbohydrates*
- *7 g fiber*
- *41 g protein*

What's in It

4 Ozs.	Cheese, mozzarella
4 Ozs.	Cheese, gouda
4 Ozs.	Salami
4 Ozs.	Proscuitto
1	Cucumber, sliced
1	Bell pepper, sliced
1	Avocado, pitted
2 Tbsp	Paleo mayonnaise
To taste	Pepper
1 Ozs.	Walnuts
1 Ozs.	Almonds

How's it Made

1. Cut all cheese and meats into bite-sized pieces and split between three plates. Divide the

cucumber, peppers, and nuts among the plates.
2. In a small bowl, scoop the avocado from the skin and add it to the bowl. Add the mayonnaise and pepper and mash until combined and creamy. Divide among plates.

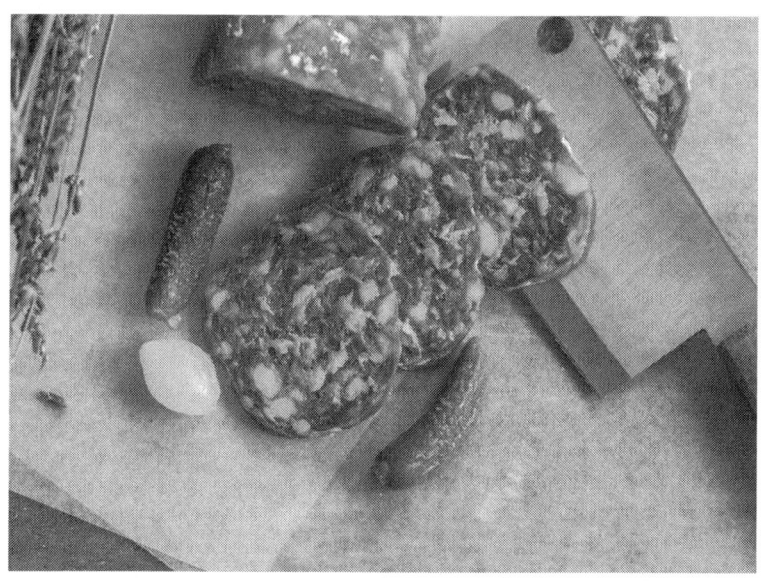

Omelet Caprese

This recipe makes 4 servings and requires about 8 minutes for cooking.

The serving size is 1 slice. It contains:

- *259 Calories*
- *20 g fat*
- *3 g total, 3 g net carbohydrates*
- *0 g fiber*
- *19 g protein*

What's in It

6	Eggs
To taste	Salt and pepper
1 Tbsp	Basil, fresh, chopped
3 Ozs	Tomatoes, cherry, halved
5 Ozs.	Cheese, mozzarella, sliced or cubed
2 Tbsp	Olive oil

How's it Made

1. In a small bowl, whisk the eggs with salt and pepper to taste. Stir in the basil.
2. In a large skillet, heat the oil over medium-high heat. Add the halved tomatoes and fry for a few minutes.

3. Pour eggs over the tomatoes and let cook for several minutes before adding cheese on top. Let cheese and egg cook for a few more minutes.
4. Turn the heat down to low and let the omelet finish cooking before transferring to a plate. Cut into quarters and serve warm.

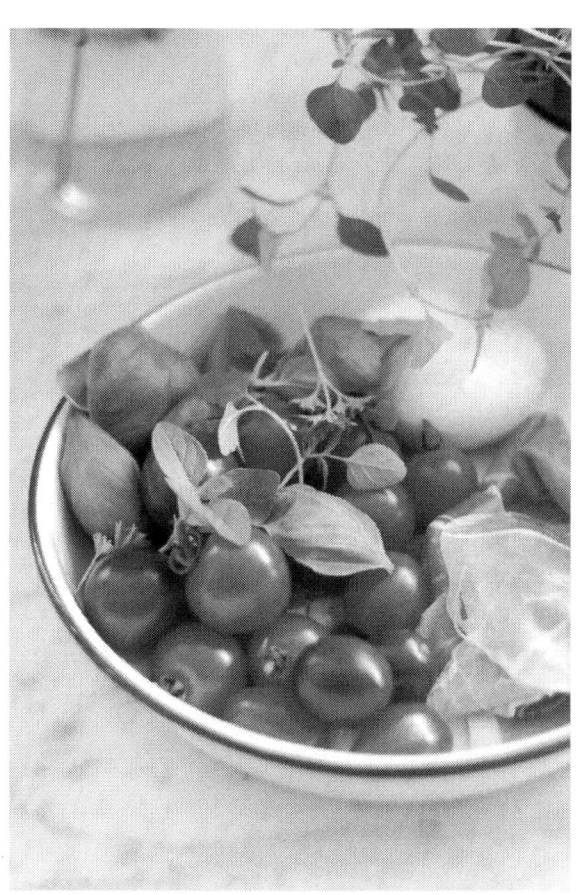

Eggs To-go

This recipe makes 6 serving and requires about 15 minutes for cooking.

The serving size is 2 cupcake liners. It contains:

- *235 Calories*
- *17 g fat*
- *3 g total, 2.5 g net carbohydrates*
- *.5 g fiber*
- *18 g protein*

What's in It

12	Eggs
4 Ozs	Bacon, cooked, chopped
1	Bell pepper, chopped
To taste	Salt and pepper

How's it Made

1. Heat your oven to 400 degree Fahrenheit. Line a muffin tin with cupcake liners.
2. In a medium bowl, mix all ingredients and pour evenly into liners.
3. Place the tin into the oven and bake for about 12 minutes or until eggs are cooked through.

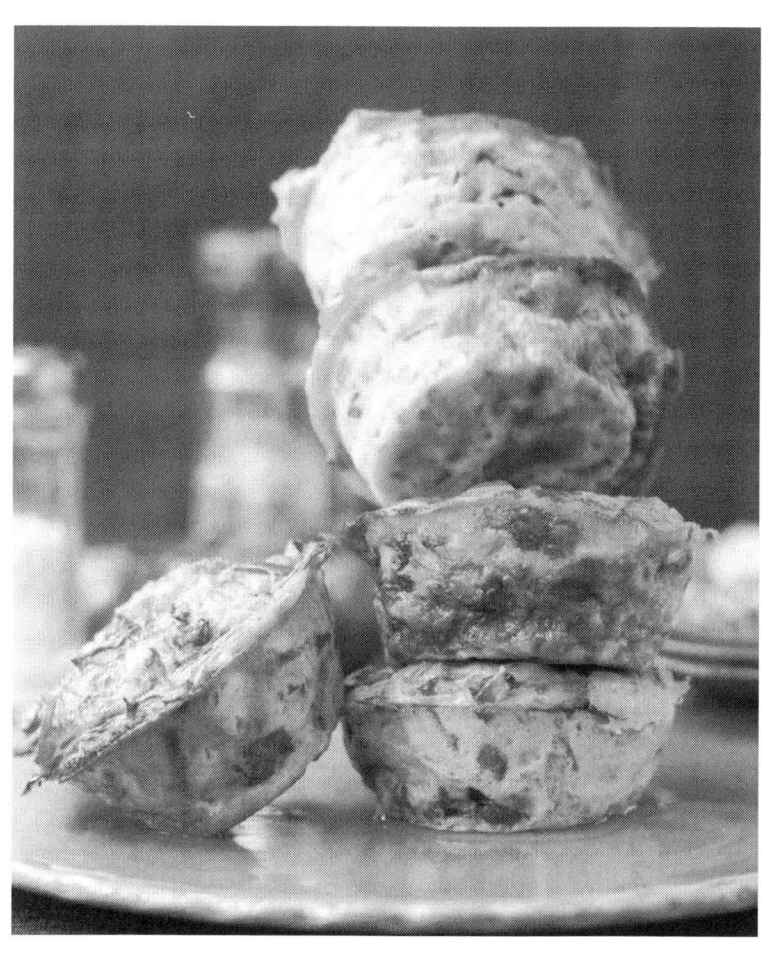

Dairy-Free Hot Chocolate

This recipe makes 1 serving and requires about 2 minutes for cooking.

The serving size is 1 mug. It contains:

- *453 Calories*
- *39 g fat*
- *14 g total, 5 g net carbohydrates*
- *9 g fiber*
- *13 g protein*

What's in It

1 Ozs	Butter
1 Tbsp	Cocoa powder
¼ tsp	Vanilla extract
1 C	Water, boiling

How's it Made

1. In a blender, combine all the ingredients and blend for about 1 minutes. Pour into a mug to serve.

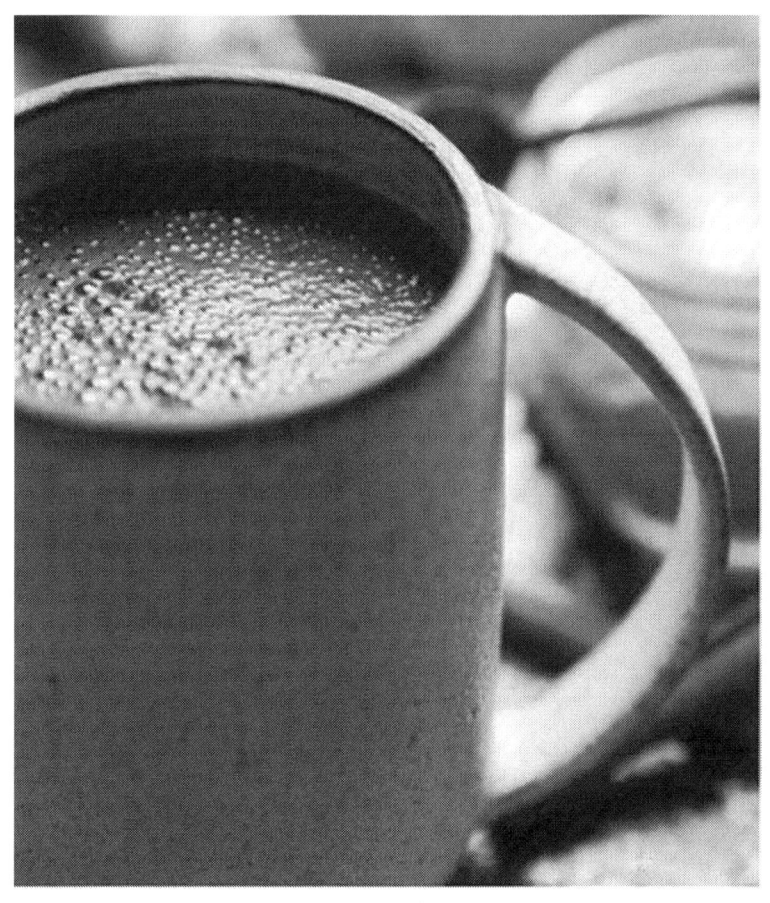

Coconut Cream and Berries

This recipe makes 1 serving and requires about 5 minutes for cooking.

The serving size is 1 bowl. It contains:

- *584 Calories*
- *57 g fat*
- *18 g total, 10 g net carbohydrates*
- *8 g fiber*
- *13 g protein*

What's in It

¼ C	Berries, frozen
4 Ozs.	Almonds
½ C	Cocont milk, full fat, unsweet
Pinch	Cinnamon

How's it Made

1. In a mixer, whip the coconut milk until creamy.
2. In a serving dish, spoon in the coconut milk cream and top with almonds and berries. Sprinkle with cinnamon.

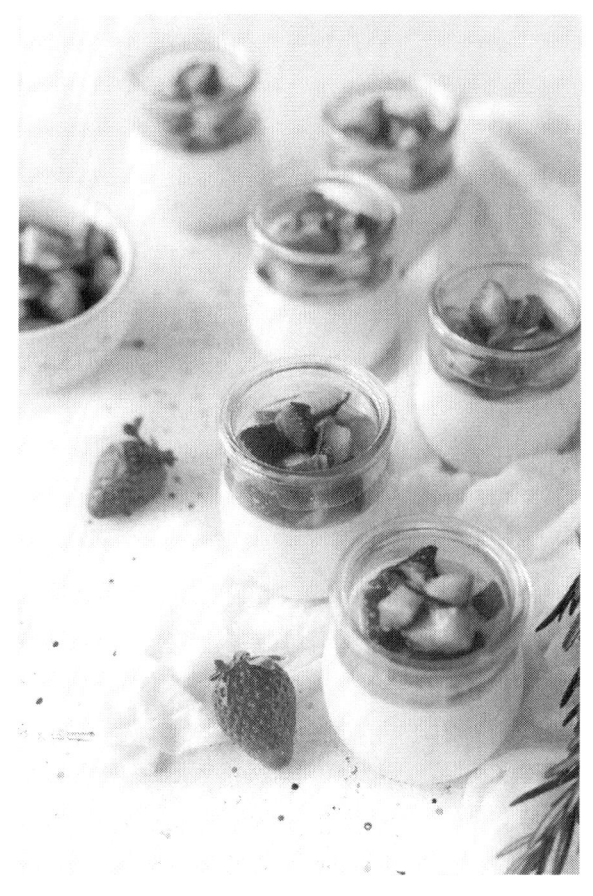

Keto Scrambled Eggs and bacon

This recipe makes 1 serving and requires about 5 minutes for cooking.

The serving size is 1 plate. It contains:

- *535 Calories*
- *48 g fat*
- *1 g total,1 g net carbohydrates*
- *0 g fiber*
- *25 g protein*

What's in It

1 Ozs	Butter
2	Eggs
To taste	Salt and pepper
2 slices	bacon

How's it Made

1. In a small bowl, whisk the eggs with salt and pepper to taste.
2. In a skillet, over medium-high heat, cook the bacon until crisp. Set aside.
3. In the same skillet, heat the butter over medium heat, if needed. Add the eggs and stir until eggs are cooked until creamy, almost completely through.

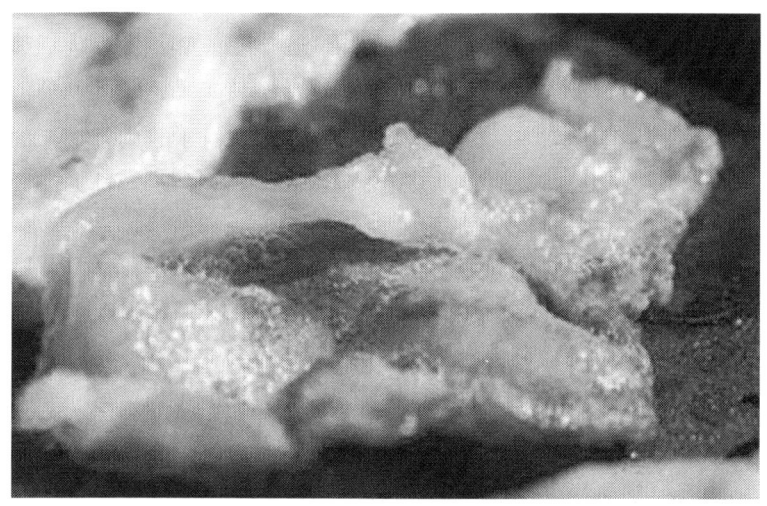

Instant, No-Cook Breakfast Options- Grab-and-go

- Sliced cheese roll-up's with chopped fresh herbs
- Lettuce leaves topped with sliced tomatoes and cheese slices
- Halved avocado topped with cured salmon slices
- Sliced meats and cheeses
- Mashed avocado with salt and pepper
- Rolled deli meats served with lettuce leaves and avocado slices
- Handful of nuts such as walnuts, hazelnuts, or almonds
- Cup of yogurt topped with nuts and fresh fruit
- Mixed nuts and seeds stirred into a cup of yogurt or milk.
- Sliced avocados topped with sliced tomatoes and cheese.

Chapter 2
Quick Ketogenic Lunches

Chicken Salad

This recipe makes 6 servings and requires about 15 minutes for cooking.

The serving size is 1 cup. It contains:

- *279 Calories*
- *19 g fat*
- *1 g total, 0 g net carbohydrates*
- *25 g fiber*
- *25 g protein*

What's in It

1.5 lbs.	Chicken breast
3	Celery stalks, diced
½ C	Paleo Mayonnaise
2 tsp	Brown mustard
½ tsp	Salt
2 Tbsp	Dill, fresh, chopped
¼ C	Pecans, chopped

How's it Made

1. On a baking sheet, line the bottom with parchment paper. Preheat the oven to 450 degrees Fahrenheit.

2. Bake the chicken for about 15 minutes or until cooked through.
3. While the chicken is baking, in a bowl, combine the celery, mayonnaise, mustard, and salt. Place in the fridge to stay cool.
4. Remove the chicken from the oven when done cooking and chop into bite-sized chunks. Allow to cool and then mix into the bowl with the other ingredients.
5. It is best to allow this to cool overnight in the fridge; however, it can be eaten immediately. Prior to serving, top with chopped dill and pecans.

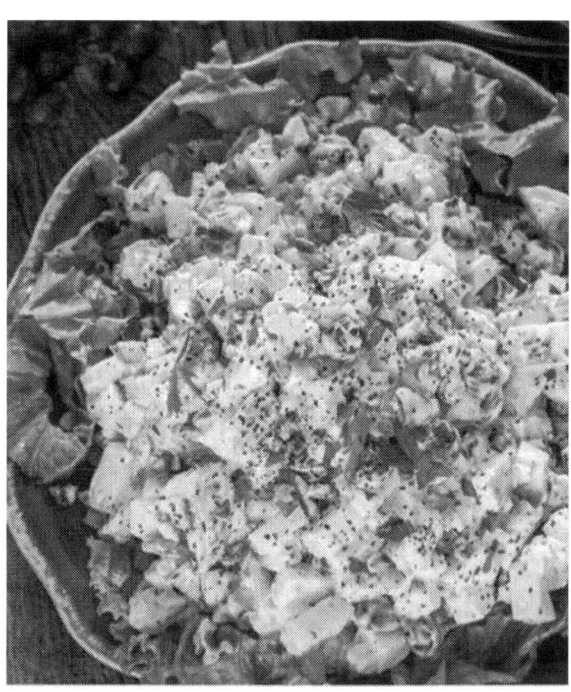

Cheese Burger with Portobello Bun

This recipe makes 6 servings and requires about 15 minutes for cooking.

The serving size is 1 cap. It contains:

- *336 Calories*
- *23 g fat*
- *6 g total, 4 g net carbohydrates*
- *2 g fiber*
- *29 g protein*

What's in It

1 lb.	Ground beef
1 Tbsp	Worcestershire sauce
1 tsp	Salt
1 tsp	Pepper
1 Tbsp	Olive oil
1 Tbsp	Avocado
6	Portobello mushroom caps, rinsed, destemmed
6	Cheddar cheese, sliced

How's it Made

1. Thoroughly mix the beef, Worcestershire, salt and pepper in a bowl. Form into 6 patties.
2. Heat the olive oil in a skillet over medium heat. Cook the mushroom caps for 3 minutes on each side. Set aside.

3. In the same skillet, add the beef patties and cook for 3 minutes on one side, 4 minutes on the other side, or until cooked through as preferred.
4. Add the cheese to the top of the burgers and cover the skillet for about 1 minute.
5. Place a beef patty on top of a mushroom cap and top with preferred toppings such as bacon, lettuce, tomato, or onion.

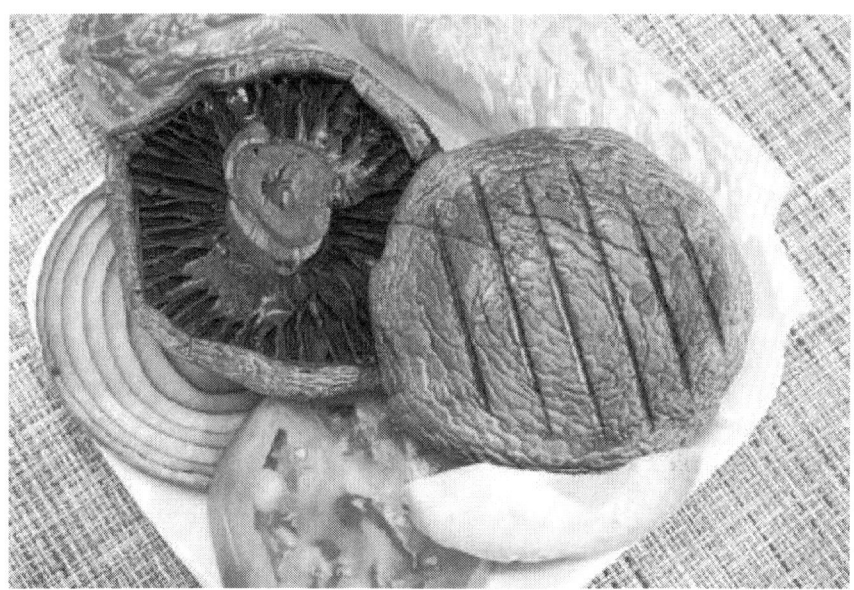

Curry Chicken Lettuce Wrap

This recipe makes 6 wraps and requires about 15 minutes for cooking.

The serving size is 3 wraps. It contains:

- *554 Calories*
- *36 g fat*
- *7 g total, 2 g net carbohydrates*
- *5 g fiber*
- *51 g protein*

What's in It

1 lb.	Chicken thighs, boneless, skinless, chopped
¼ C	Onion, minced
2 cloves	Garlic, minced
2 tsp	Curry powder
1 ½ tsp	Salt
1 tsp	Pepper
3 Tbsp	Butter
1 C	Cauliflower rice
6 leaves	Lettuce
¼ C	Sour cream or plain, unsweet coconut yogurt

How's it Made

1. In a large skillet, heat 2 tablespoons butter over medium heat. Add the onion and sauté until browned.
2. Mix in the chicken, garlic and salt. Cook for about 8 minutes.
3. Add the remaining tablespoon of butter, curry and rice and cook until combined.
4. Spread out lettuce leaves and spoon in mixture evenly, topping with a spoonful of cream or yogurt.

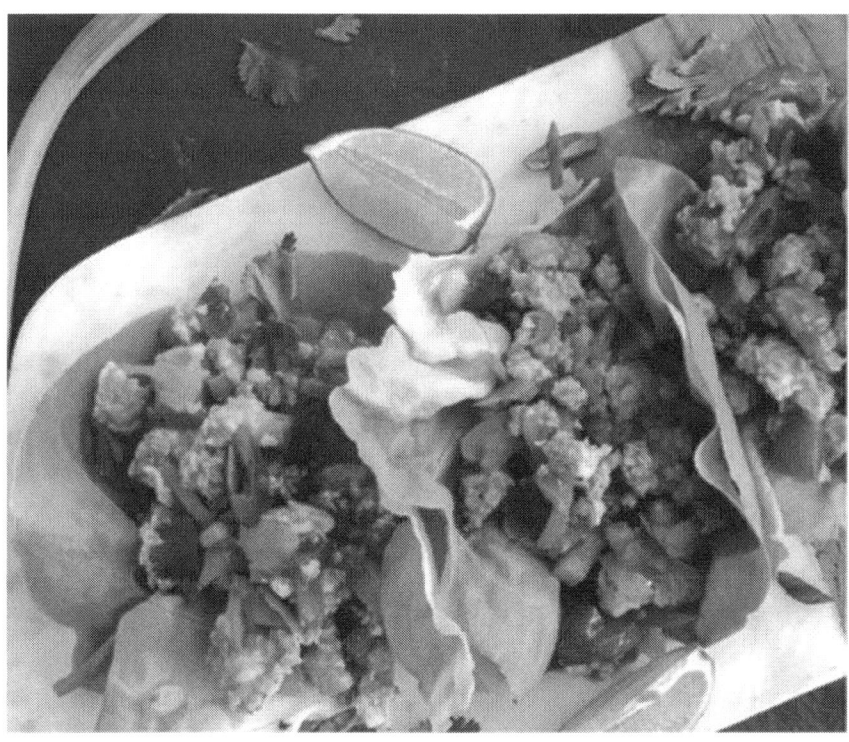

Avocado Salad

This recipe makes 2 halves and requires about 5 minutes for cooking.

The serving size is 1 half. It contains:

- *697 Calories*
- *64 g fat*
- *27 g total, 11 g net carbohydrates*
- *16 g fiber*
- *12 g protein*

What's in It

2	Tomatoes, chopped
2/3 C	Feta cheese, crumbled
1/3 C	Red onion, chopped
2 Tbsp	Parsley, fresh, chopped
2 Tbsp	Olive oil
1 Tbsp	Red wine vinegar
1 tsp	Oregano, fresh, chopped
To taste	Salt and pepper
2	Avocados

How's it Made

1. Halve the avocados and remove the pits. Do not remove the avocado from the skin. Set aside.
2. In a small bowl, combine all the ingredients except the avocado. Spoon the mixture evenly

into the two avocados where the pits were previously.

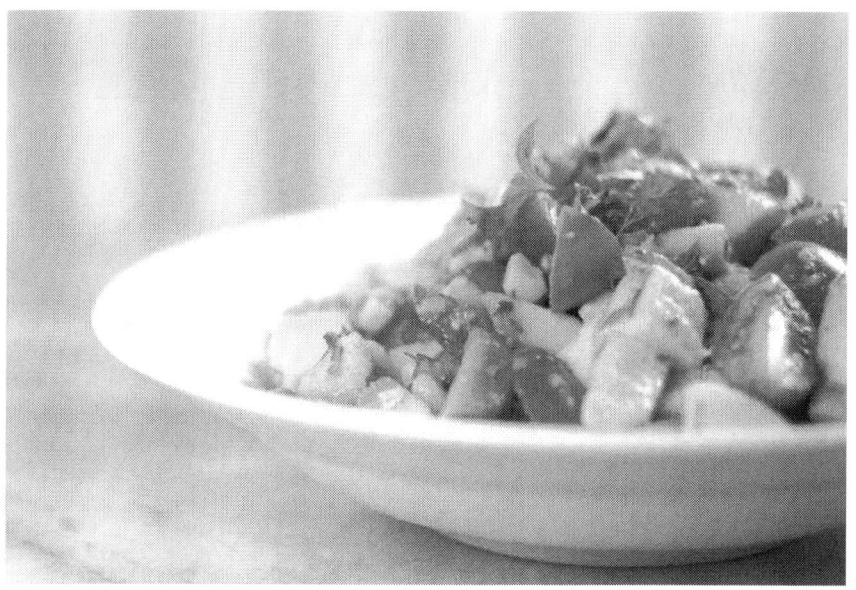

Turkey Wrap

This recipe makes 3 wraps and requires about 5 minutes for cooking.

The serving size is 1 wrap. It contains:

- *279 Calories*
- *20 g fat*
- *8 g total, 5 g net carbohydrates*
- *3 g fiber*
- *18 g protein*

What's in It

3 slices	Turkey meat, deli
3 slices	Provolone cheese
3 slices	Tomato
3 leaves	Lettuce
½	Avocado, mashed
3 Tbsp	Paleo mayonnaise

How's it Made

1. In a bowl, mix the mayonnaise and avocado. Set aside.
2. On a plate, place the lettuce leaves down. Spread 1/3 the mayonnaise mixture on the leaf, then place the turkey, tomato, and cheese on each leaf. Roll the lettuce to hold all the ingredients together.

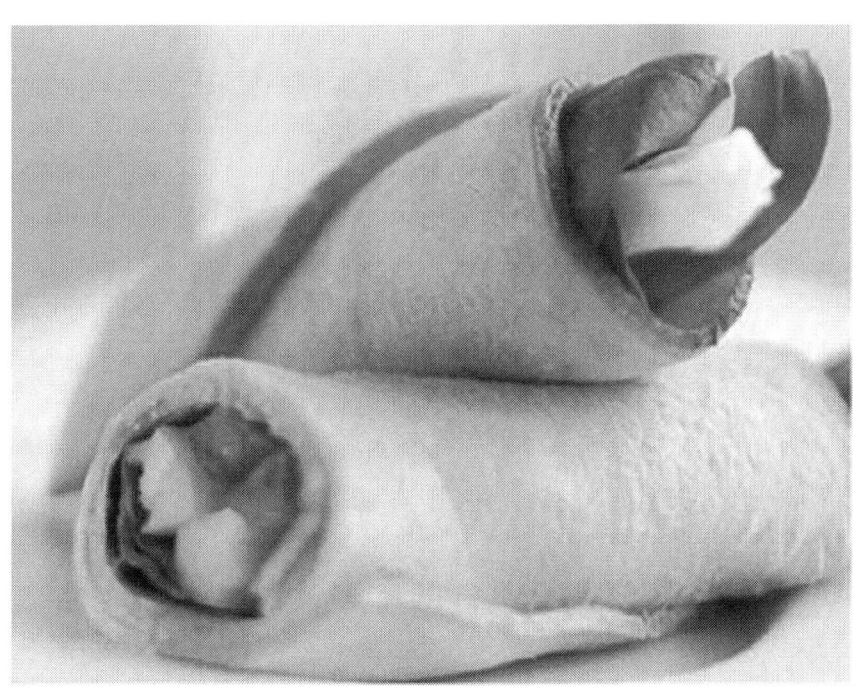

Spicy Shrimp Salad

This recipe makes 2 salads and requires about 15 minutes for cooking.

The serving size is 1 salad. It contains:

- *727 Calories*
- *24 g fat*
- *27 g total, 24 g net carbohydrates*
- *3 g fiber*
- *99 g protein*

What's in It

1 Tbsp	Olive oil
4 cloves	Garlic, minced
½ lb	Shrimp, raw, cleaned
½ tsp	Cumin
½ tsp	Old Bay seasoning
¼ tsp	Chili pepper powder
¼ tsp	Cayenne pepper powder
3 Tbsp	Tahini
½ C	Apple cider vinegar
2 Tbsp	Water
1 ½ tsp	Ginger, fresh, minced
2 Tbsp	Honey
2 tsp	Lime juice
To taste	Salt and pepper

How's it Made

1. In a skillet,
2. heat the oil over medium-high heat. Add the 3 cloves of the garlic and shrimp and seasonings; cayenne, chili, Old Bay, and cumin. Cook for several minutes on each side until pink throughout. Remove from heat and chop.
3. In a small bowl, toss the lime juice and avocado.
4. In the two serving bowls, divide the salad greens and cucumber. Top with avocado and shrimp.
5. In another small bowl, whisk the tahini, vinegar, water, ginger, honey, lime juice, and garlic until combined. Add salt and pepper, if desired. Drizzle dressing over the top of the salad bowls.

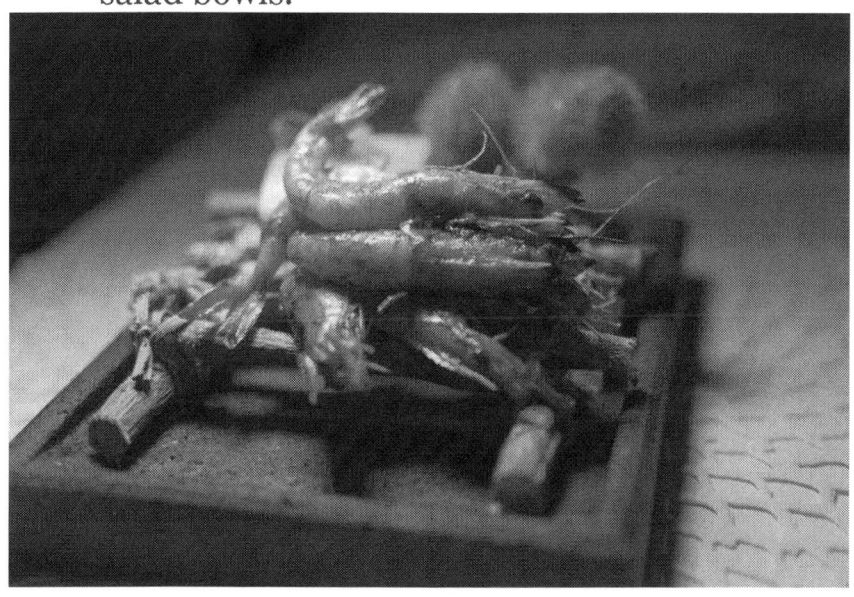

Smoked Tuna Boat

This recipe makes 6 servings and requires about 5 minutes for cooking.

The serving size is 2 pickle boats. It contains:

- *254 Calories*
- *14 g fat*
- *2 g total, 2 g net carbohydrates*
- *0 g fiber*
- *29 g protein*

What's in It

6 spears	Pickles, Dill, whole
2 cans	Tuna, albacore, 6 ozs cans
1 can	Tuna, smoked, 6 ozs can
1/3 C	Paleo mayonnaise
1 Tbsp	Onion, dried or ½ tsp powder
¼ tsp	Garlic powder
¼ tsp	Pepper

How's it Made

1. Halve the pickles lengthwise and scoop out the insides and seeds to make a "boat." Set the insides aside and use for another recipe.
2. In a small bowl, combine the remaining ingredients until well mixed. Divide evenly between the pickle halves. Best refrigerated

for a few hours and served cold but can be eaten immediately.

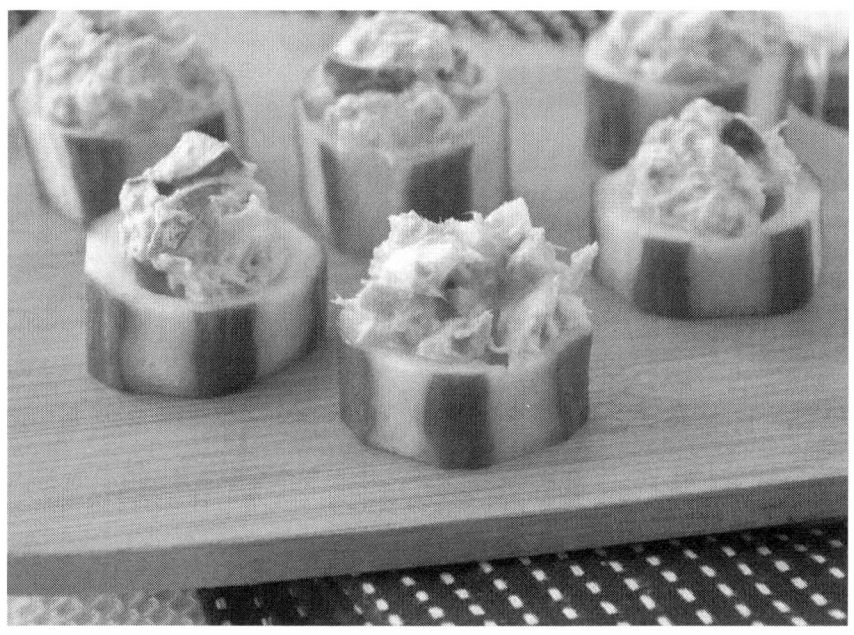

Cauliflower and Broccoli Salad

This recipe makes 7 servings and requires about 15 minutes for cooking.

The serving size is 1 cup. It contains:

- *324 Calories*
- *32 g fat*
- *5 g total, 3 g net carbohydrates*
- *2 g fiber*
- *7 g protein*

What's in It

8 Ozs	Broccoli florets, chopped
8 Ozs	Cauliflower florets, chopped
2 Ozs	Red pepper, diced
4 Ozs	Cheddar cheese, diced
1/3 lbs	Bacon, cooked, crumbled
2 Tbsp	Red onion, chopped
¾ C	Paleo mayonnaise
¾ C	Plain Greek yogurt
2 Tbsp	Sugar or sweetener
1 Tbsp	Lemon juice, fresh

How's it Made

1. In a large bowl combine the broccoli, cauliflower, red pepper, cheese, and onion.

2. In a separate bowl, stir together the mayonnaise, yogurt, sweetener and lemon juice. Adjust seasoning as needed.
3. Toss the salad and dressing together and top with the crumbled bacon bits.

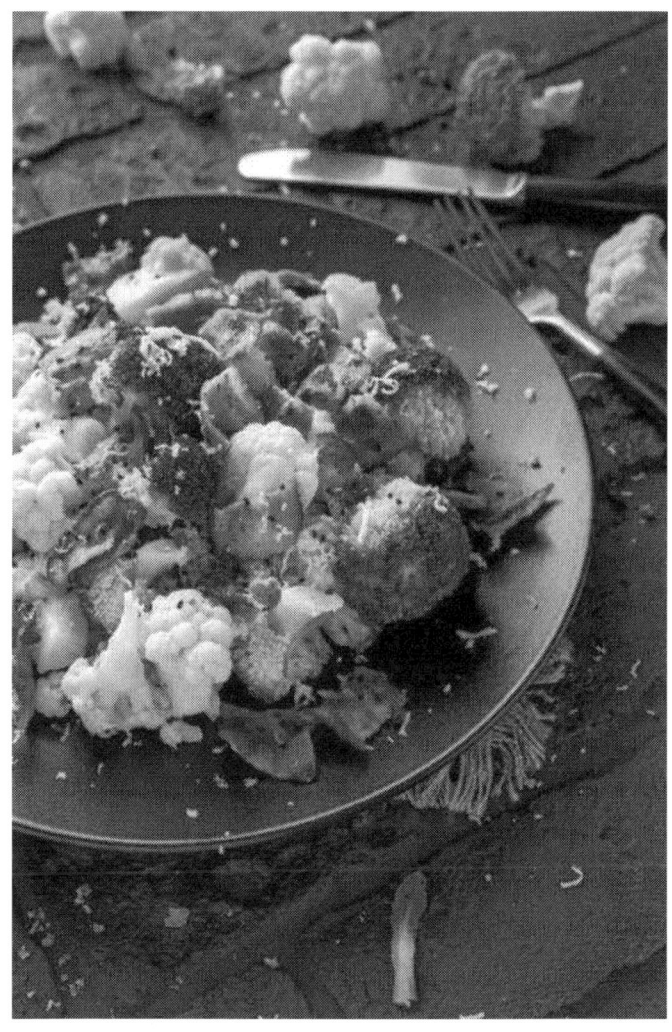

Italian Salad

This recipe makes 2 servings and requires about 5 minutes for cooking.

The serving size is 2 cups. It contains:

- *748 Calories*
- *51 g fat*
- *58 g total, 40 g net carbohydrates*
- *18 g fiber*
- *28 g protein*

What's in It

4 C	Lettuce, shredded
2	Tomatoes, diced
1 C	Olives, Italian, mixed
¼	Red onion, sliced
¼ C	Banana peppers, pickled, sliced
6 Ozs	Meat, Italian, diced
2 ½ Tbsp	Olive oil
2 Tbsp	Red wine vinegar
1 Tbsp	Italian seasoning
To taste	Salt and pepper

How's it Made

1. In a small bowl mix the oil, vinegar, seasoning, and salt and pepper. Set aside.

2. In a large bowl, mix the lettuce, tomatoes, olives, onion, peppers, and meat. Drizzle with the oil and vinegar dressing.

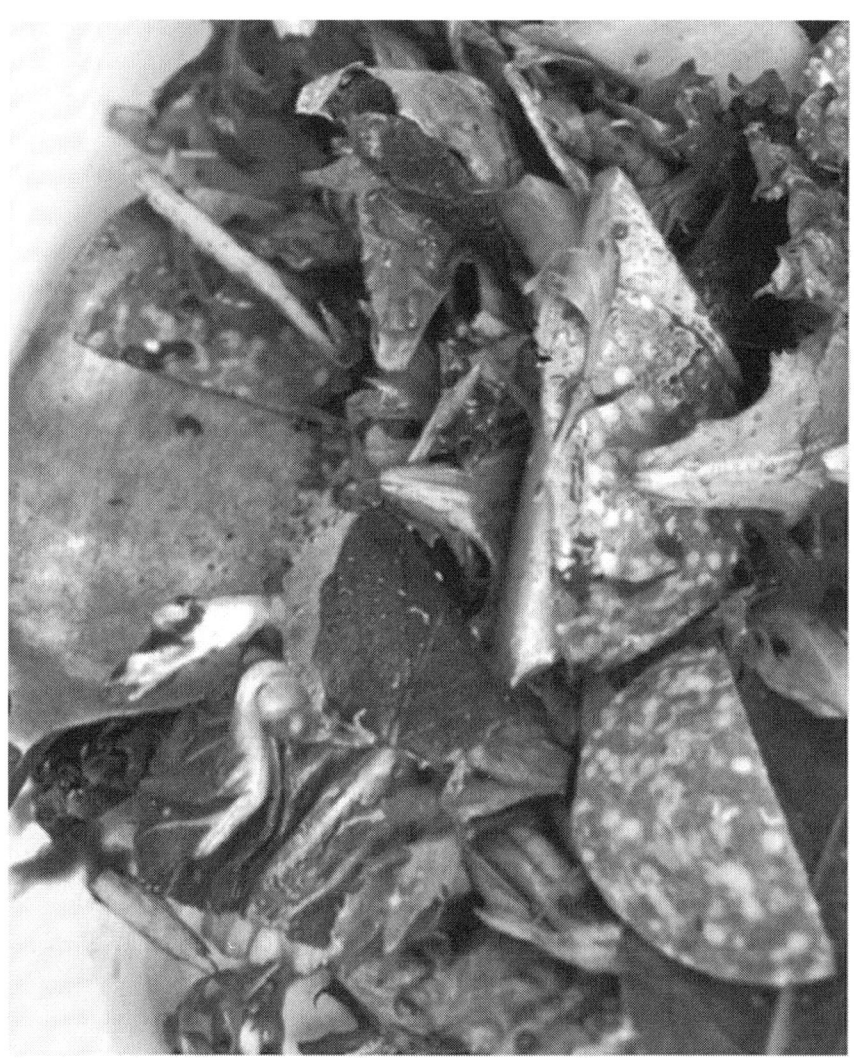

Creamy Cilantro Salad

This recipe makes 3 servings and requires about 10 minutes for cooking.

The serving size is 2 cups. It contains:

- *821 Calories*
- *32 g fat*
- *7 g total, 5 g net carbohydrates*
- *2 g fiber*
- *119 g protein*

What's in It

¼ C	Paleo mayonnaise
3 Tbsp	Cilantro, fresh, minced
1 Tbsp	Water
2 tsp	Lemon juice, fresh
1	Lemon, zest
¼ tsp	Garlic powder
½ tsp	Salt
6 C	Lettuce, chopped
6 Ozs	Shrimp, cooked
4 Ozs	Chicken breast, cooked, sliced
2	Eggs, boiled, halved
¼ C	Bacon, cooked, crumbled
1 C	Tomatoes, sliced
½ C	Cilantro, fresh, chopped
1	Scallion, sliced

How's it Made

1. In a small bowl whisk together the mayonnaise, minced cilantro, water, lemon juice, zest, garlic powder and salt. Set aside.
2. In a large bowl, layer lettuce on the bottom and top with shrimp, chicken, eggs, bacon, and tomatoes. Sprinkle cilantro and scallions on top.
3. Drizzle with cilantro dressing before serving.

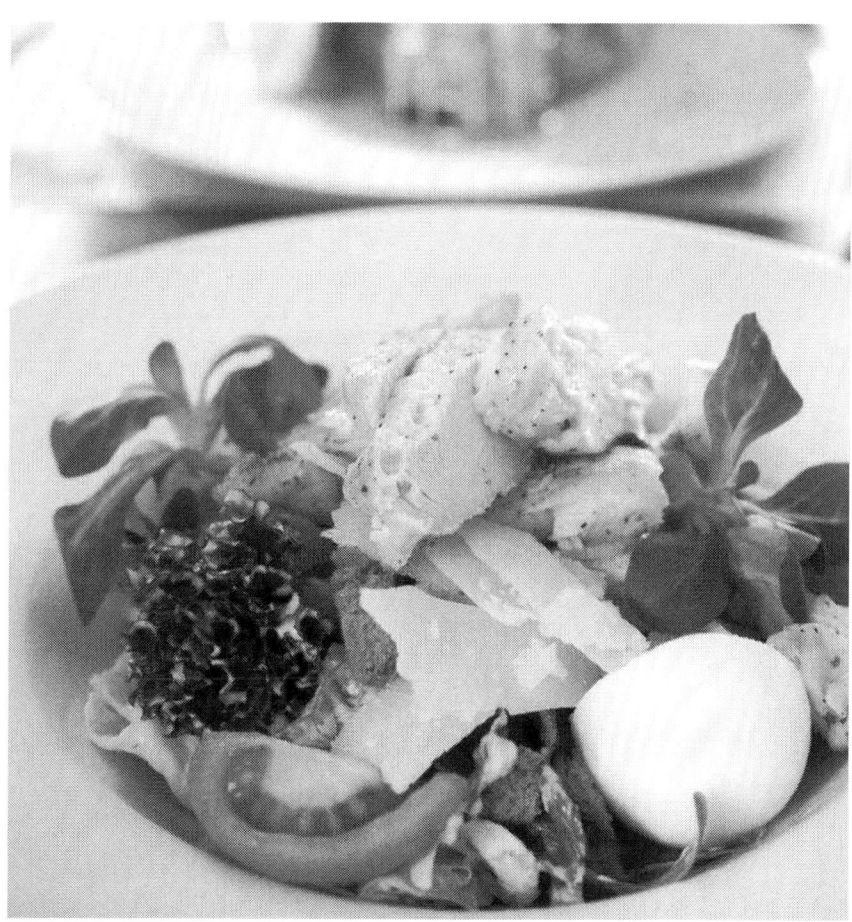

Mega Wedge Salad

This recipe makes 2 servings and requires about 15 minutes for cooking.

The serving size is 1 wedge. It contains:

- *849 Calories*
- *39 g fat*
- *50 g total, 42 g net carbohydrates*
- *8 g fiber*
- *76 g protein*

What's in It

¼ C	Greek yogurt, plain
3 Tbsp	Sour cream
1 Tbsp	Paleo mayonnaise
3 Tbsp	Milk
Dash	Worcestershire sauce
¼ C	Bleu cheese, crumbled
2 tsp	Balsamic vinegar
To taste	Salt and pepper
1	Iceberg lettuce, quartered
1/3 C	Bacon, cooked, crumbled
4	Eggs, hard boiled, chopped
10	Tomatoes, grape, halved

How's it Made

1. Whisk the yogurt, cream, mayonnaise, milk, Worcestershire, and bleu cheese in a small bowl and set aside.
2. Place two of the iceberg wedges on two plates with the cut sides facing up. Add the remaining ingredients and drizzle with the creamy dressing. Consider adding some extra bleu cheese crumbles on top for a garnish.

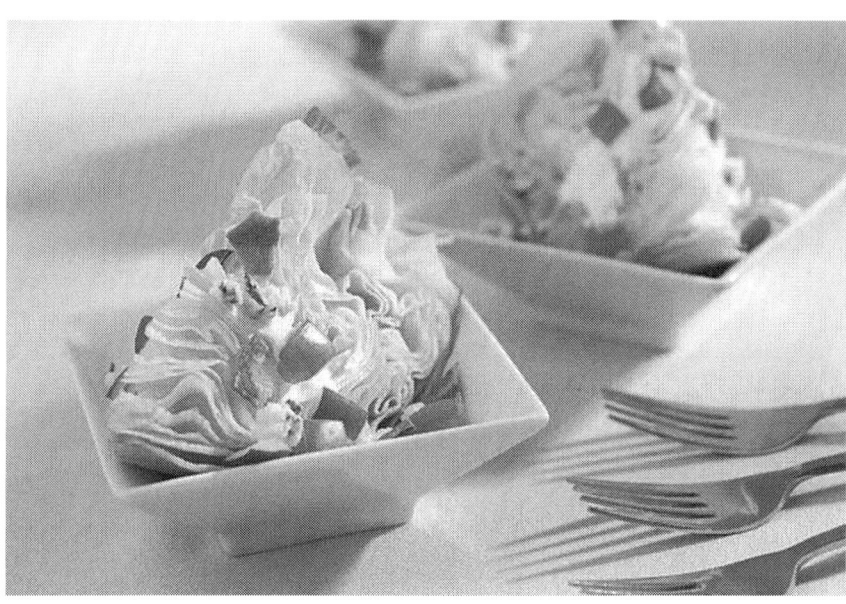

Meatball Sub

This recipe makes 2 servings and requires about 1 minute for cooking.

The serving size is 1 sub. It contains:

- *612 Calories*
- *44 g fat*
- *20 g total, 17 g net carbohydrates*
- *3 g fiber*
- *52 g protein*

What's in It

2 Slices	Provolone
6	Meatballs, precooked
2 Tbsp	Tomato sauce
To taste	Salt and pepper

How's it Made

1. In a microwave safe dish, warm up the meatballs and sauce, if desired, for about 30 seconds.
2. On a plate, place the cheese slices flat and then add 3 meatballs to each slice. Evenly split the sauce between the two subs. Sprinkle with salt and pepper, if desired.

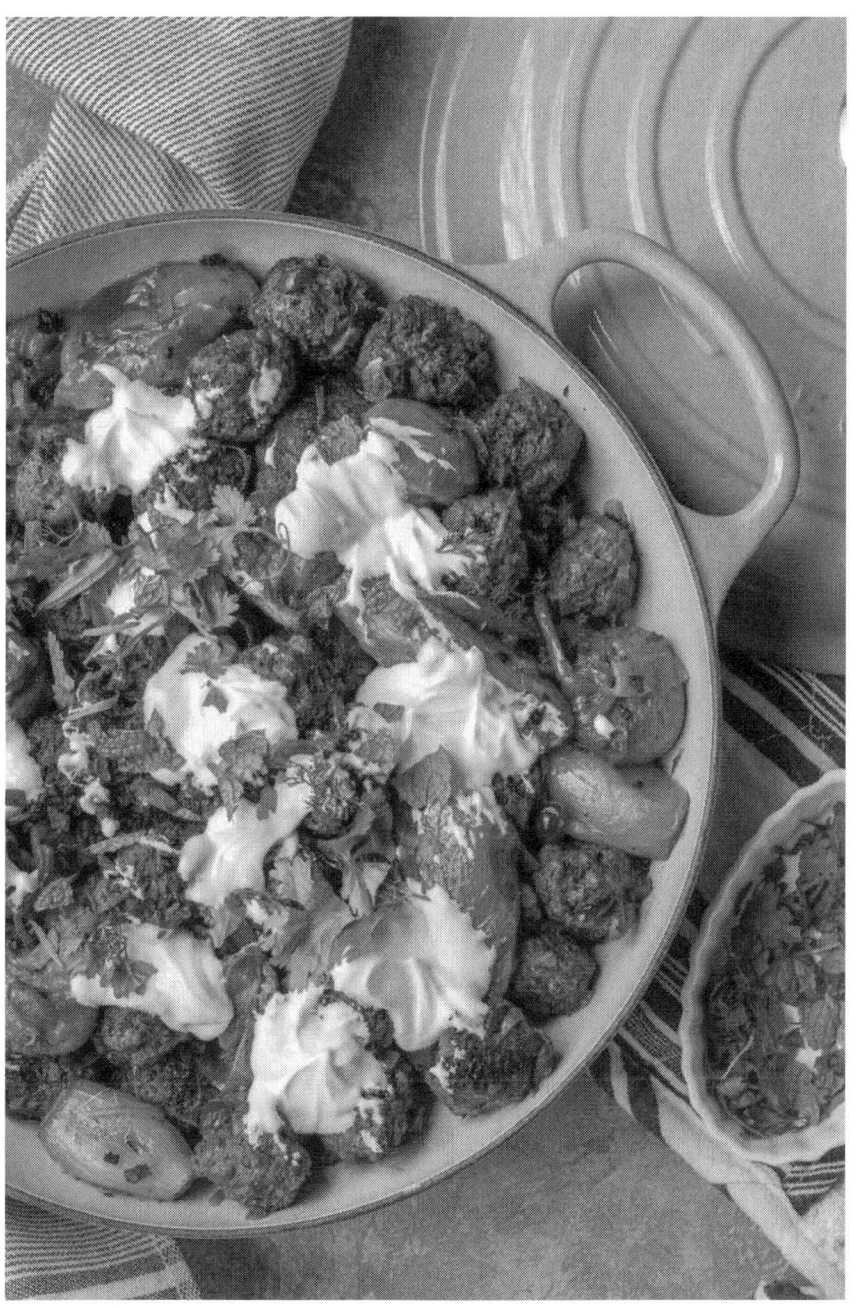

Monte Cristo Sandwich

This recipe makes 2 sandwiches and requires about 15 minutes for cooking.

The serving size is 1 sandwich. It contains:

- *1006 Calories*
- *68 g fat*
- *27 g total, 20 g net carbohydrates*
- *7 g fiber*
- *70 g protein*

What's in It

½ Tbsp	Olive oil
4 Ozs	Cream cheese
4	Eggs
1 tsp	Cinnamon
2 Tbsp	Coconut flour
1 tsp	Sugar or preferred sweetener
4 slices	Turkey
4 slices	Ham
2 C	Swiss cheese, shredded

How's it Made

1. Heat up oil in a skillet over medium heat.
2. In a small bowl, whisk the cream cheese, eggs, cinnamon, flour, and sweetener until combined.

3. Pour ¼ of the mixture onto the skillet in a circle and cook for about 1 minute, flip and cook on the other side until cooked through. Repeat until all the mix is used.
4. Lower the heat to medium-low and place 1 pancake on the skillet. Top with 1 slice of turkey, 1 slice of ham, and a sprinkle of cheese. Cover the skillet and cook for about 30 seconds until the cheese is melted. Remove from heat and top with 1 pancake to make a sandwich. Garnish with a sprinkle of cheese, if desired. These are best eaten warm, either fresh or reheated in a microwave.

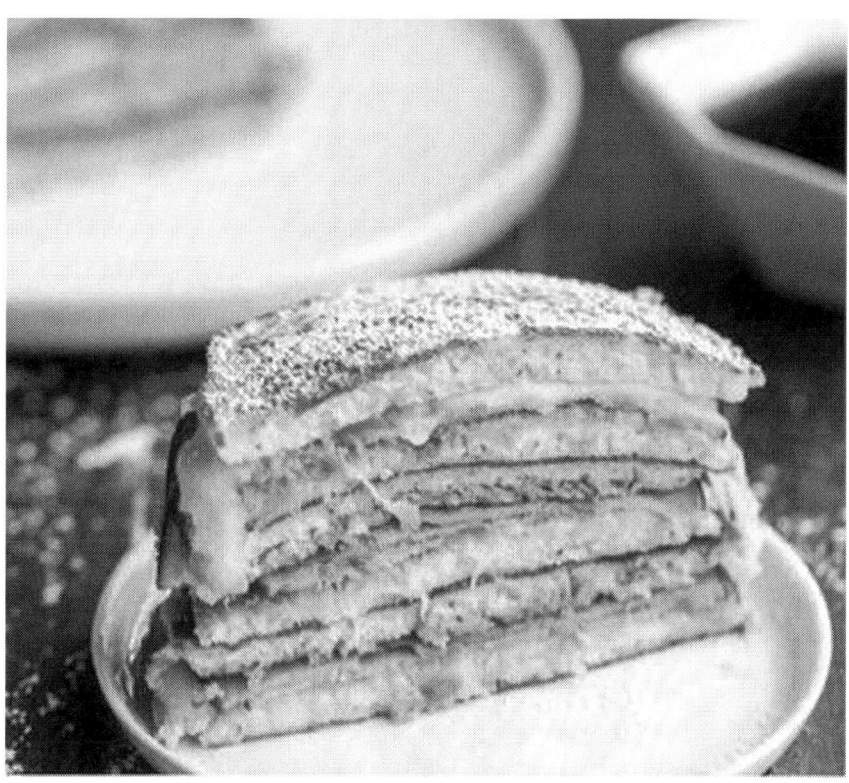

Spinach and Shrimp Salad

This recipe makes 1 serving and requires about 5 minutes for cooking.

The serving size is 2 cups. It contains:

- *564 Calories*
- *46 g fat*
- *4 g total, 2 g net carbohydrates*
- *2 g fiber*
- *31 g protein*

What's in It

7 Ozs	Shrimp, fresh, cleaned
1 Tbsp	Butter
2 C	Spinach, fresh
¼ C	Olives
2 Tbsp	Olive oil
To taste	Salt and pepper
Dash	Cayenne pepper

How's it Made

1. In a skillet, heat the butter over medium heat. Add the shrimp and cook until pink, turning often. Remove from heat.
2. In a bowl, combine the remaining ingredients. Top with warm shrimp.

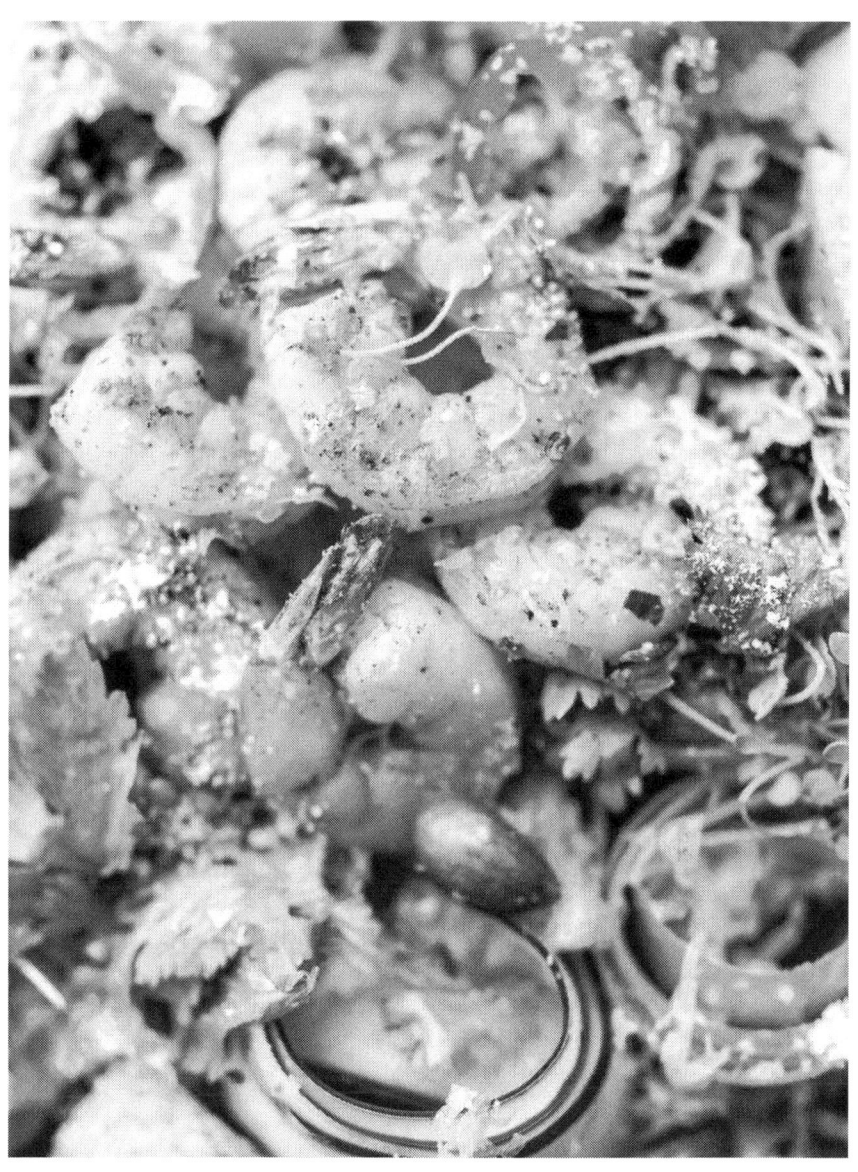

Cheese Quesadilla

This recipe makes 1 serving and requires about 13 minutes for cooking.

The serving size is 2 quesadillas. It contains:

- *715 Calories*
- *63 g fat*
- *5 g total, 4 g net carbohydrates*
- *1 g fiber*
- *37 g protein*

What's in It

2	Eggs
2	Eggs, whites only
6 Ozs	Cream cheese
1 ½ tsp	Psyllium, powder or other natural thickener
1 Tbsp	Almond flour
½ tsp	Salt
5 Ozs	Cheese, jack, shredded
1 Ozs	Spinach, fresh
1 Tbsp	Olive oil

How's it Made

1. Heat your oven to 400 degrees Fahrenheit. Line a baking tray with parchment paper.

2. In a mixer, add the eggs and egg whites and beat until light. Mix in the cream cheese and mix until creamy.
3. In a small bowl, whisk flour, psyllium powder, and salt. Slowly add it to the mixing bowl while mixing slow. Once combined, allow the mixture to thicken for a few minutes.
4. Pour the batter on to the tray and spread out evenly with a spatula. Place in the oven and bake for about 6 minutes or until the edges are browned.
5. Remove from the oven and cut into desired pieces.
6. In a skillet, heat the oil over medium heat. Place one tortilla piece in the skillet, top with half the cheese and half the spinach. Place another tortilla on top. Flip over after 1 minute and allow it to cook on the other side, until the cheese melts. Repeat with the remaining tortillas, cheese, and spinach.

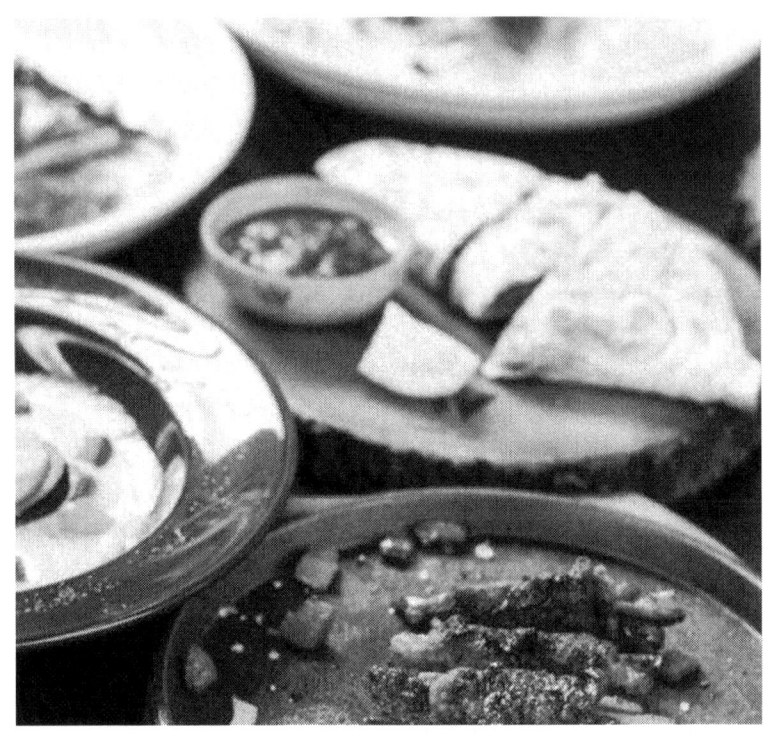

Meatballs with Pimento Cheese

This recipe makes 4 servings and requires about 15 minutes for cooking.

The serving size is 5-8 meatballs. It contains:

- *616 Calories*
- *34 g fat*
- *15 g total, 13 g net carbohydrates*
- *2 g fiber*
- *62 g protein*

What's in It

1 ½ lbs	Beef, ground
1	Egg
To taste	Salt and pepper
2 Tbsp	Butter
4 Ozs	Cheese, cheddar, shredded
Pinch	Cayenne
1 Tbsp	Mustard, Dijon
1 tsp	Paprika
4 Tbsp	Pimentos
1/3 C	Paleo mayonnaise

How's it Made

1. In a large bowl, combine the mayonnaise, pimentos, paprika, mustard, cayenne, and cheddar until thoroughly mixed. Let sit for 2 minutes.

2. While the cheese is setting, in a skillet over medium heat, warm the oil.
3. Stir in the beef, salt and pepper until combined.
4. Separate the mixture into even balls and add them to the hot skillet. Stir gently often to evenly cook throughout. Serve over a cup of fresh spinach or eat alone while hot.

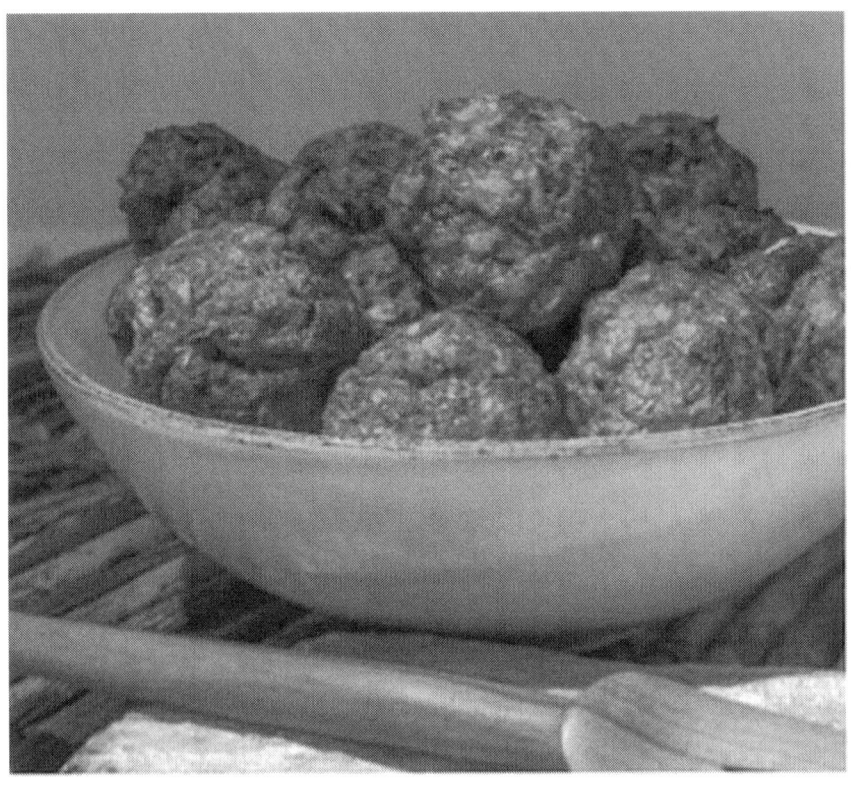

Halloumi Cheese with Mushrooms and Olives

This recipe makes 4 servings and requires about 10 minutes for cooking.

The serving size is 1/4 cheese steak. It contains:

- *609 Calories*
- *52 g fat*
- *17 g total, 12 g net carbohydrates*
- *3 g fiber*
- *19 g protein*

What's in It

2/3 lb	Halloumi cheese
2/3 lb	Mushrooms, rinsed, sliced
3 Ozs	Butter
10	Olives
To taste	Salt and pepper
½ C	Paleo mayonnaise

How's it Made

1. In a large skillet, heat the butter over medium heat and add the mushrooms. Cook for about 3 minutes or until golden. Sprinkle with salt and pepper as desired.
2. Make room for the cheese in the middle of the pan and cook the cheese for 2 minutes on each side while continuing to stir the mushrooms.

3. Remove from heat, cut the cheese in half and serve each half with olives.

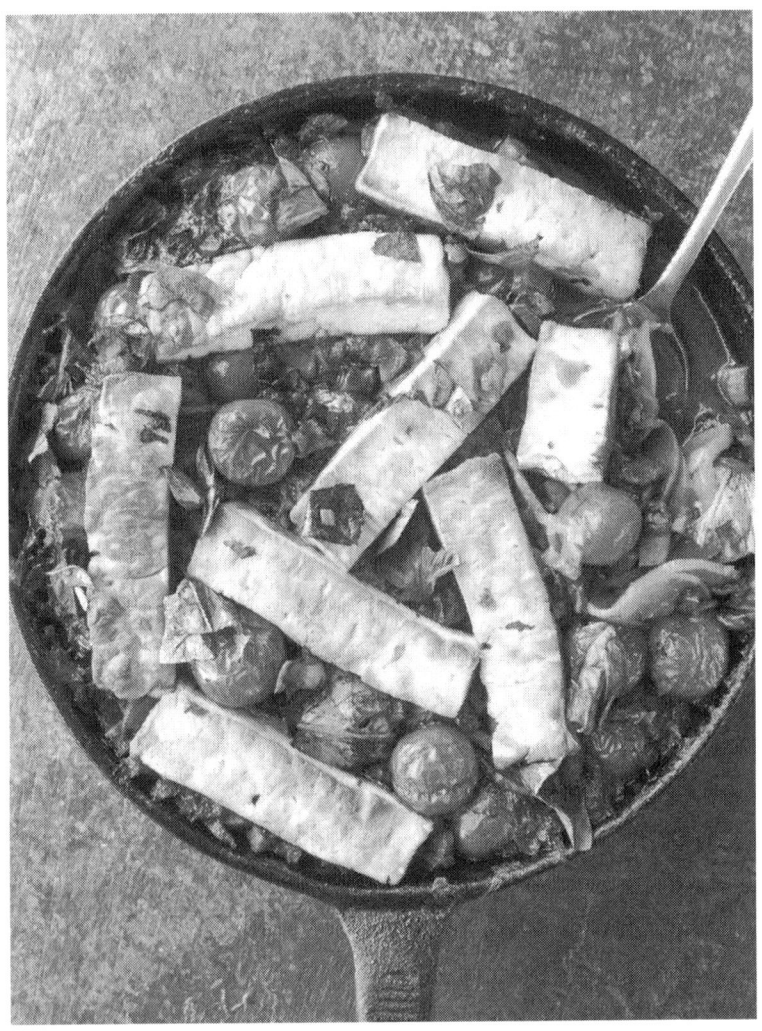

Spinach and Salmon

This recipe makes 2 servings and requires about 7 minutes for cooking.

The serving size is 1 salmon steak. It contains:

- *279 Calories*
- *19 g fat*
- *1 g total, 0 g net carbohydrates*
- *25 g fiber*
- *25 g protein*

What's in It

¾ lb	Salmon, cut in half
2 Tbsp	Butter
½	Bell pepper, sliced
2 Oz	Spinach, fresh
To taste	Salt and pepper

How's it Made

1. In a skillet, heat the butter over medium heat. Add the salmon and cook for about 3 minutes on each side. Sprinkle with salt and pepper. Lower the heat.
2. On two serving plates, divide the spinach evenly among the plates and top with one salmon steak. Garnish with bell pepper slices.

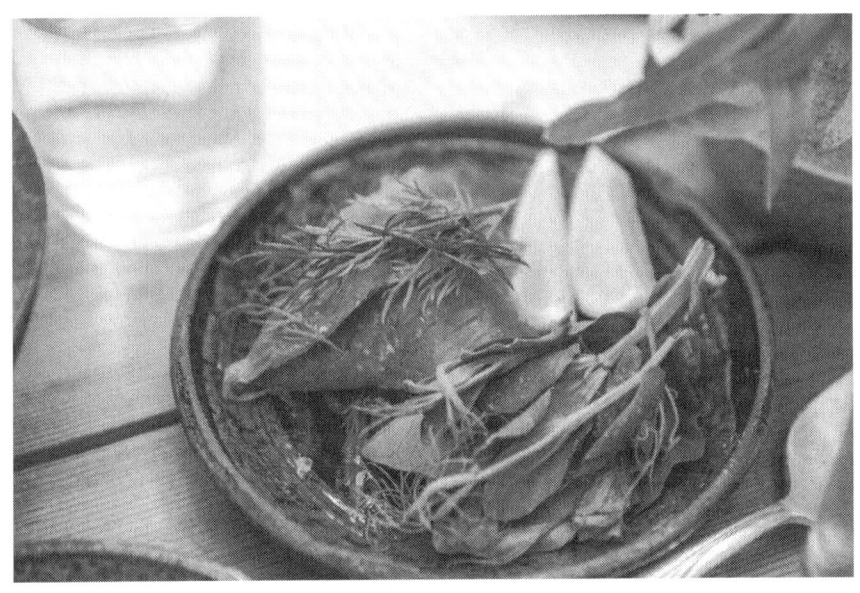

Ranch Pork Skewer with Salsa Verde Sauce

This recipe makes 4 servings and requires about 15 minutes for cooking.

The serving size is 2 skewers and ¼ of the sauce. It contains:

- *659 Calories*
- *61 g fat*
- *2 g total, 1.5 g net carbohydrates*
- *.5 g fiber*
- *27 g protein*

What's in It

1 lb	Pork shoulder, sliced
½ Tbsp	Ranch seasoning
1 tsp	Salt
1 Tbsp	Butter
6 Tbsp	Parsley, fresh, chopped
3 Tbsp	Basil, fresh, chopped
2 cloves	Garlic, minced
1/2	Lemon, juiced
3 Tbsp	Capers
2/3 C	Olive oil
½ tsp	Pepper

How's it Made

1. In a blender or food processor, add the salt, pepper, olive oil, lemon juice, capers, garlic, basil and parsley and mix until combined. Set aside.
2. In a medium bowl, place the pork inside and sprinkle with ranch seasoning and salt. Skewer each seasoned pork slice.
3. In a skillet, heat the butter over medium-high heat and add the pork skewers. Cook 3 minutes on each side or until cooked through.
4. Place 2 skewers on a plate and top with ¼ of the sauce.

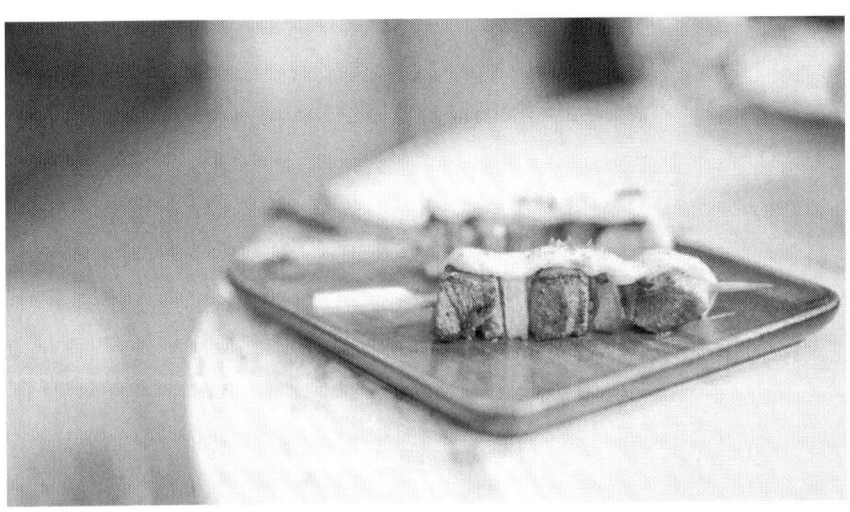

Instant, No-Cook Lunch Options- Grab-and-go

- Smoked salmon with sliced tomatoes and olives
- Turkey deli meat with sliced avocado and fresh spinach
- Canned artichokes, drained, dipped in mayonnaise or Greek yogurt
- Bleu cheese slices with prosciutto
- Salami with brie cheese and a handful of macadamia nuts
- Sauerkraut and roast beef deli meat
- Ham deli meat rolled around cucumber slices, bell pepper slices, and avocado slices
- Canned tuna with sliced vegetables
- Beef jerky with a handful of nuts
- Avocado sprinkled with salt and served with smoked salmon or prosciutto

Chapter 3
Quick Ketogenic Dinners

Chili Chicken Thighs

This recipe makes 4 servings and requires about 15 minutes for cooking.

The serving size is 1 serving. It contains:

- *467 Calories*
- *21 g fat*
- *1 g total, .5 g net carbohydrates*
- *.5 g fiber*
- *66 g protein*

What's in It

2 lbs.	Chicken thighs, boneless
1 Tbsp	Olive oil
1 Tbsp	Chili powder
To taste	Salt and pepper
To taste	Cilantro, fresh, minced
As desired	Lime wedge, for garnish

How's it Made

1. On a baking sheet, place the chicken and rub all over with the oil. Add the spices and rub in.
2. Heat your oven to 350 degrees Fahrenheit.

3. Place the chicken in the hot oven and cook for about 15 minutes, or until fully cooked.
4. When ready to serve, add cilantro and a lime wedge.

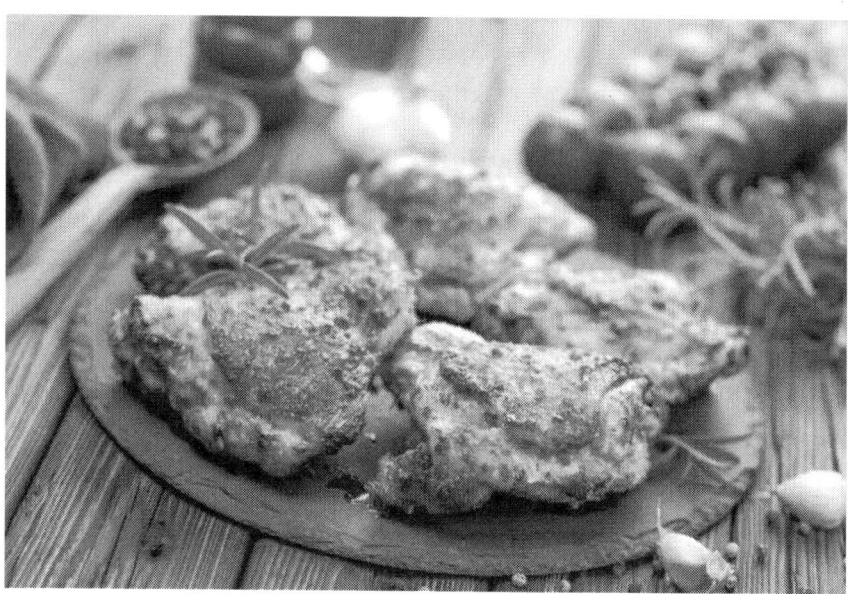

Garlic Dipped Grilled Chicken Skewers

This recipe makes 2 servings and requires about 15 minutes for cooking.

The serving size is 1 serving. It contains:

- *1671 Calories*
- *158 g fat*
- *26 g total, 21 g net carbohydrates*
- *5 g fiber*
- *53 g protein*

What's in It

1 lbs.	Chicken breast, cubed
1	Onion, chopped
2	Bell peppers, chopped
1	Zucchini
1 head	Garlic, peeled
2 tsp	Salt
¼ C	Lemon juice, fresh
1 1/2 C	Olive oil

How's it Made

1. Create the marinade and garlic sauce by blending the garlic, ½ of the lemon juice, and ½ cup of the olive oil until well combined and the garlic is well chopped. Slowly add the remaining juice and ½ cup of oil, alternating

until the sauce begins to combine well and turn into a stiff mixture.
2. Place ½ the mixture aside for dipping and stir in the remaining ½ cup of oil and 1 teaspoon of salt to the other half.
3. In the bowl of garlic sauce that received the extra oil and salt, mix in the chicken and vegetables.
4. Preheat the grill to high heat.
5. Place the marinated chicken and vegetables on to skewers, alternating the ingredients and trying to keep each skewer even. Place the skewers on the grill and cook on high until the chicken is cooked through, about 10 minutes. Serve along with the remaining garlic sauce for dipping.

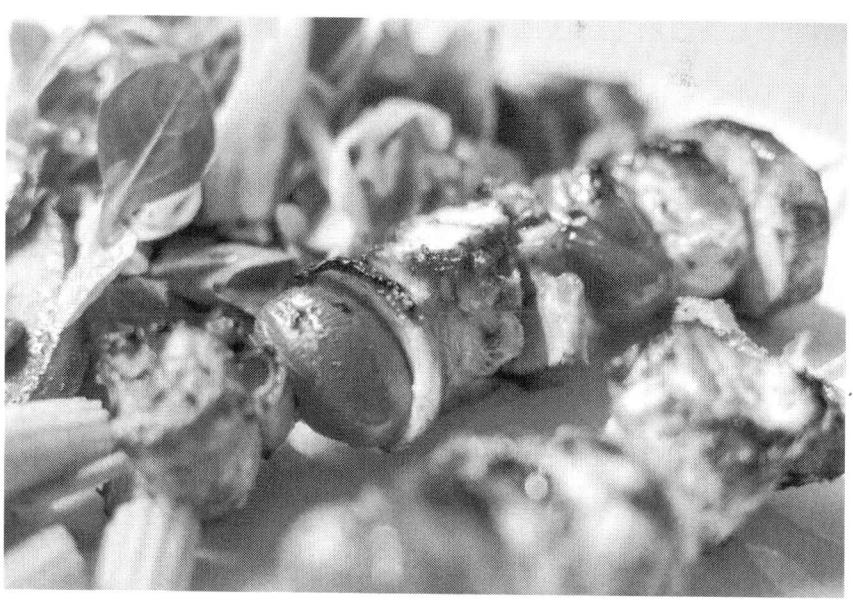

Bacon Burgers on a Lettuce "Bun"

This recipe makes 4 servings and requires about 9 minutes for cooking.

The serving size is 2 burgers. It contains:

- *558 Calories*
- *24 g fat*
- *1 g total, 1 g net carbohydrates*
- *0 g fiber*
- *79 g protein*

What's in It

2 lbs.	Beef, ground
2	Eggs
4 slices	Bacon, raw, diced
½ tsp	Chili powder
8 leaves	Lettuce
As desired	Tomato, onion, etc.

How's it Made

1. In a large bowl combine all the ingredients except for the lettuce and desired garnishes. Do not over mix.
2. Separate the meat into even balls and create patties by pressing down on the balls.

3. On the grill or a skillet over medium heat, cook the burger patties for about 4 minutes on one side and 3 minutes on the other.
4. Removed from the grill and serve on lettuce leaves and topped with your preferred toppings.

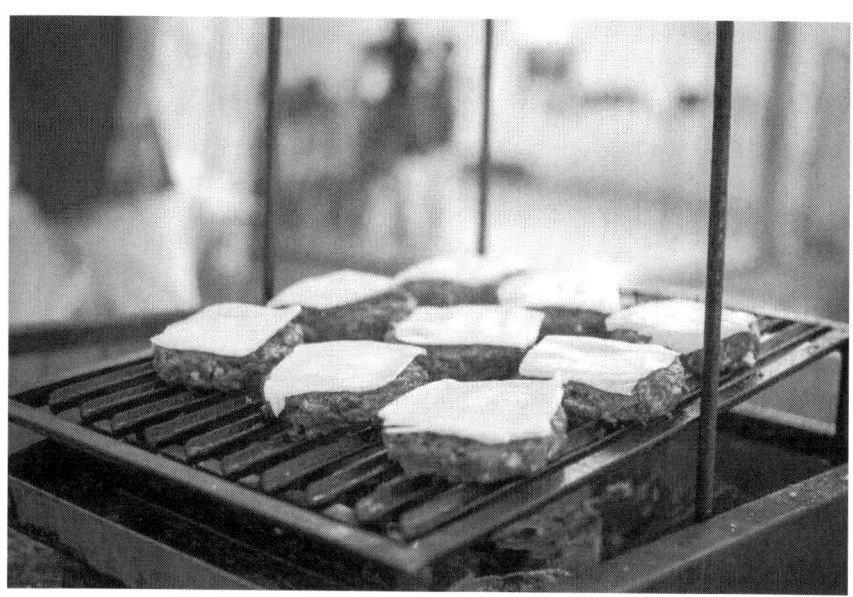

Thai Chili and Lemon Halibut

This recipe makes 4 servings and requires about 15 minutes for cooking.

The serving size is 1/2 piece. It contains:

- *467 Calories*
- *21 g fat*
- *1 g total, .5 g net carbohydrates*
- *.5 g fiber*
- *66 g protein*

What's in It

4 C	Spinach
2	Halibut steaks, 11 ozs ea.
1/2	Lemon, juiced
To taste	Salt and pepper
To taste	Paprika
½	Lemon, sliced
As desired	Scallions, chopped
1	Thai chili, deseeded, sliced
1 C	Tomatoes, cherry, halved
2 Tbsp	Olive oil

How's it Made

1. Heat your oven to 400 degrees Fahrenheit.
2. Tear off 2 equal squares of tin foil and divide the spinach amongst them.
3. If your halibut still has the middle bone and membrane, remove this with a knife. This will

split the halibut steak in half, resulting in four pieces of fish.
4. Place two pieces of halibut or one full steak in one Foil Square and the remaining fish in the other square. Pour ½ the lemon juice over one foil and the rest on the other.
5. Sprinkle the seasonings on each and fish steak and top with a slice of lemon. On top of the lemon place scallions, chili, and tomatoes. Drizzle with ½ tablespoon on each fish piece.
6. Close the foil around the fish and bake on a tray for about 12 minutes.
7. Remove from the foil before serving. Drizzle the juices on top and remove the skins, if preferred.

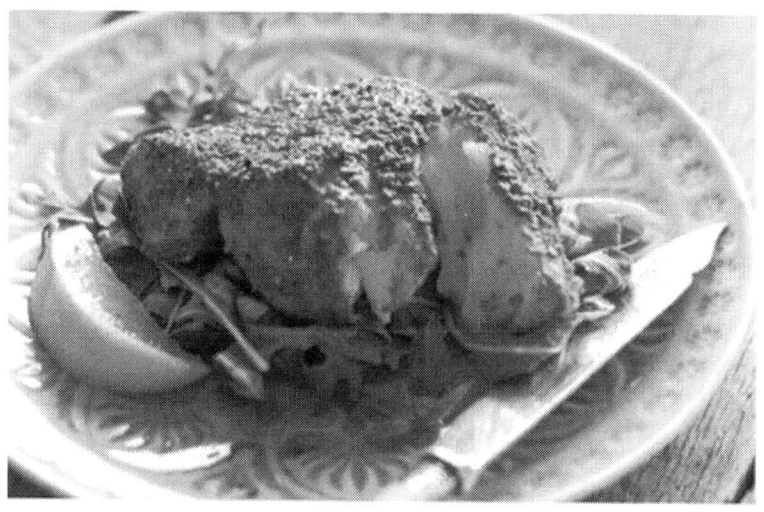

Salmon patties with Avocado Sauce

This recipe makes 12 patties and requires about 15 minutes for cooking.

The serving size is 3 patties. It contains:

- *532 Calories*
- *39 g fat*
- *8 g total, 4 g net carbohydrates*
- *4 g fiber*
- *40 g protein*

What's in It

1 lb	Salmon, canned
2	Eggs
¼ C	Almond flour
3 Tbsp	Parsley, fresh, chopped
1 Tbsp	Dill, fresh, chopped
1 Tbsp	Lemon juice
1	Onion, diced
2 cloves	Garlic, chopped
1 tsp	Paprika
½ tsp	Cumin
½ tsp	Turmeric
To taste	Salt and pepper
2 Tbsp	Butter
1	Avocado, pit removed
¼ C	Paleo mayonnaise
1 Tbsp	Lime juice

How's it Made

1. In a large bowl, combine the salmon, eggs, flour, 1 tablespoon of parsley, dill, lemon juice, onion, 1 clove of garlic, paprika, cumin, turmeric and salt and pepper. Do not over mix.
2. Scoop out the mixture and form into 12 even patties.
3. In a skillet, heat the butter and cook each patty for 4 minutes on one side and about 3 minutes on the other side.
4. While the patties are cooking, in a blender, place the avocado, mayonnaise, lime juice, 1 clove of garlic, 1 tablespoon of parsley, and salt and pepper and mix until smooth.
5. Place 3 patties over a bed of lettuce and drizzle with avocado sauce.

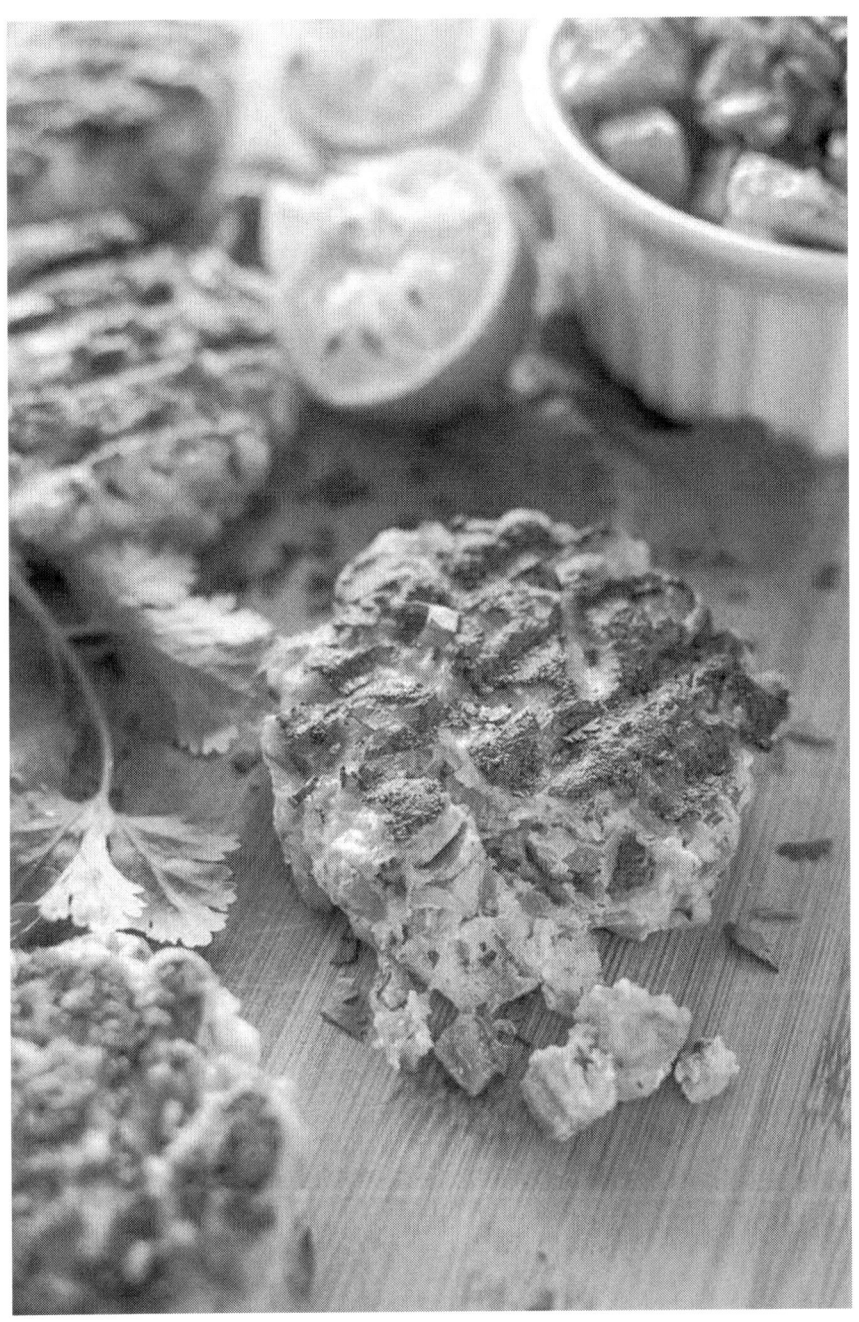

Chicken "Noodle" Soup

This recipe makes 4 servings and requires about 15 minutes for cooking.

The serving size is 1 cup. It contains:

- *204 Calories*
- *14 g fat*
- *4 g total, 3 g net carbohydrates*
- *1 g fiber*
- *14 g protein*

What's in It

1 Tbsp	Butter
½	Onion, diced
6 C	Chicken broth
1 C	Water
1 lbs	Chicken, precooked, chopped
1 tsp	Basil, dried
1 tsp	Oregano, dried
1 tsp	Parsley, dried
To taste	Salt and pepper
2	Squash

How's it Made

1. Over medium heat, melt the butter in a large stockpot. Place the onion in the pot and cook for a few minutes until clear.

2. Pour in the broth and water. Add the chicken and herbs and stir to combine. Bring to a boil and then reduce to a simmer for about 5 minutes covered.
3. Using a mandolin slicer or spiralizer, cut the squash into strips. When the simmering is complete, add the squash "noodles" and cook for 7 minutes, uncovered.

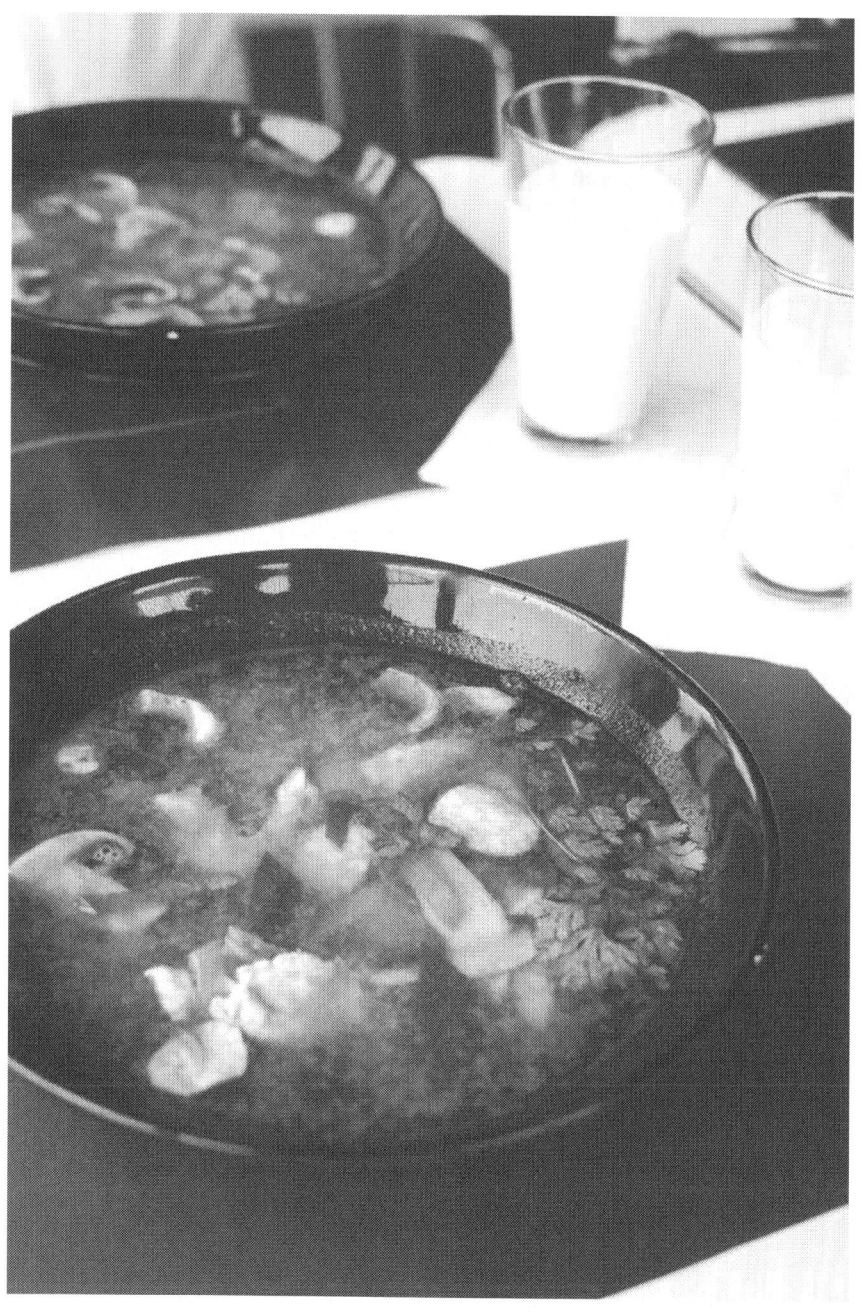

Beef Steak and Onions

This recipe makes 4 steaks and requires about 15 minutes for cooking.

The serving size is 2 beef steaks. It contains:

- *423 Calories*
- *18 g fat*
- *10 g total, 8 g net carbohydrates*
- *2 g fiber*
- *53 g protein*

What's in It

4 Cubes	Beef steak
2	Onions, sliced
1 ¼ Tbsp	Adobo seasoning
2 Tbsp	Vinegar
1 Tbsp	Olive oil

How's it Made

1. In a skillet, heat the oil over medium-high heat. Add the onions and sauté until browned. Lower the heat to medium.
2. On each side of the steak cubes, sprinkle 1 tablespoon of adobo seasoning and then 1 tablespoon of vinegar.
3. In the skillet with the onions, add the remaining ¼ tablespoon of adobo seasoning

and 1 Tablespoon of vinegar and stir to combine.
4. Create a hole in the middle of the onions and add the steak. Use the onions to cover the steak and cook until the edges are browned.
5. Flip the steak and cook another few minutes until it is cooked through.

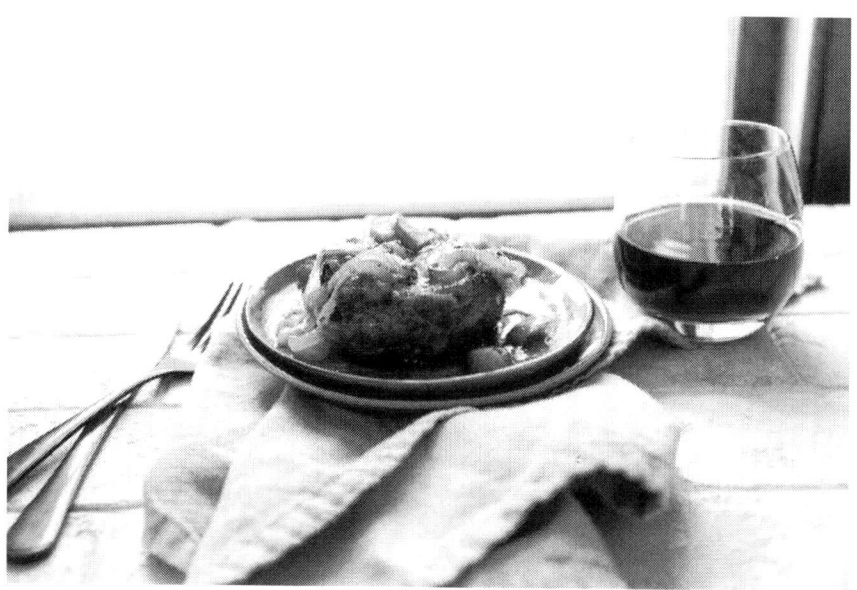

Beef Lettuce Wraps

This recipe makes 4 servings and requires about 15 minutes for cooking.

The serving size is 1 wrap. It contains:

- *467 Calories*
- *21 g fat*
- *1 g total, .5 g net carbohydrates*
- *.5 g fiber*
- *66 g protein*

What's in It

2 lbs.	Beef, lean, ground
2 C	Beef broth
3 cloves	Garlic, chopped
1/3 C	Lime juice, fresh
3 Tbsp	Fish sauce
2/3 C	Cilantro, fresh, chopped
2/3 C	Mint, fresh, chopped
As desired	Lettuce for serving

How's it Made

1. In a skillet, over medium-high heat, brown the beef, breaking it up with a spoon, for about 7 minutes.

2. Once brown, pour in the broth and stir. Simmer for about 6 minutes or until most of the broth is gone.
3. In a small bowl, mix the garlic, lime juice, and fish sauce. Lay lettuce leaves out.
4. Once the broth is evaporated, add the lime garlic sauce and simmer for another 2 minutes. Stir in the herbs then remove from heat.
5. Add the beef to the lettuce leaves for serving.

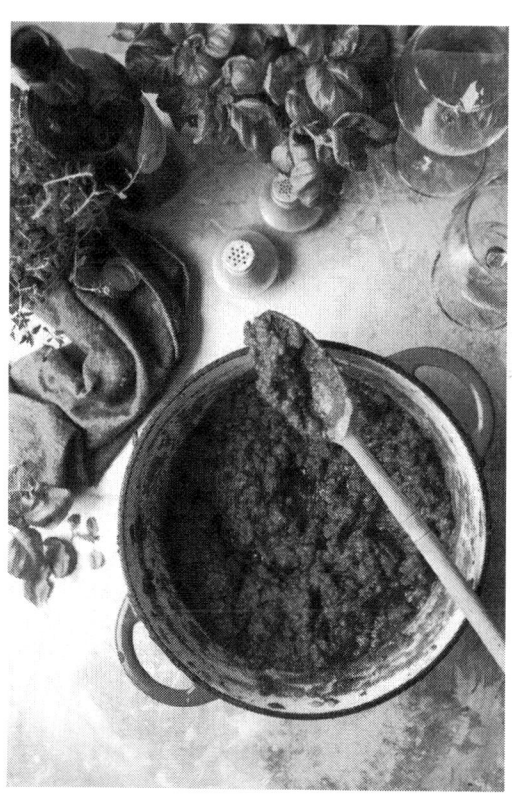

Broccoli Beef

This recipe makes 2 servings and requires about 10 minutes for cooking.

The serving size is ½ bowl. It contains:

- *382 Calories*
- *22 g fat*
- *9 g total, 6 g net carbohydrates*
- *3 g fiber*
- *39 g protein*

What's in It

2 C	Broccoli florets
½ lb	Beef, precooked
3 cloves	Garlic, minced
1 tsp	Ginger, fresh, grated
2 Tbsp	Tamari sauce
2 Tbsp	Olive oil

How's it Made

1. In a large skillet, heat about 2 tablespoons of oil and stir in the broccoli.
2. When broccoli reaches your desired crispness stir in the beef. Cook for about 2 minutes.
3. Mix in the garlic, ginger and tamari sauce and remove from heat.

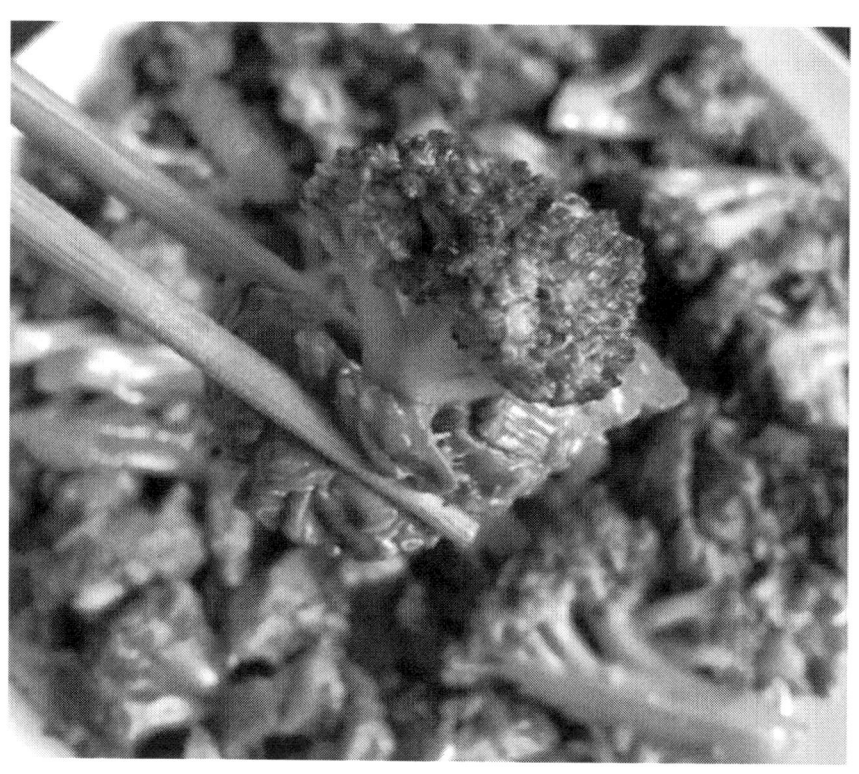

Lobster Roll

This recipe makes 4 servings and requires about 5 minutes for cooking.

The serving size is 2 rolls. It contains:

- *600 Calories*
- *37 g fat*
- *22 g total, 19 g net carbohydrates*
- *3 g fiber*
- *44 g protein*

What's in It

2 C	Lobster meat, cooked, chopped
1 ½ C	Cauliflower florets, cooked, cooled
½ C	Paleo mayonnaise
1 tsp	Tarragon, fresh, chopped
8 leaves	Romaine lettuce
½ C	Tomatoes, chopped
½ C	Bacon, cooked, chopped

How's it Made

1. In a bowl, stir the lobster and cauliflower together with the mayonnaise and tarragon until creamy.
2. Lay out the lettuce leaves and spoon the lobster mixture into each of them evenly.

Topped with chopped tomatoes and bacon and serve.

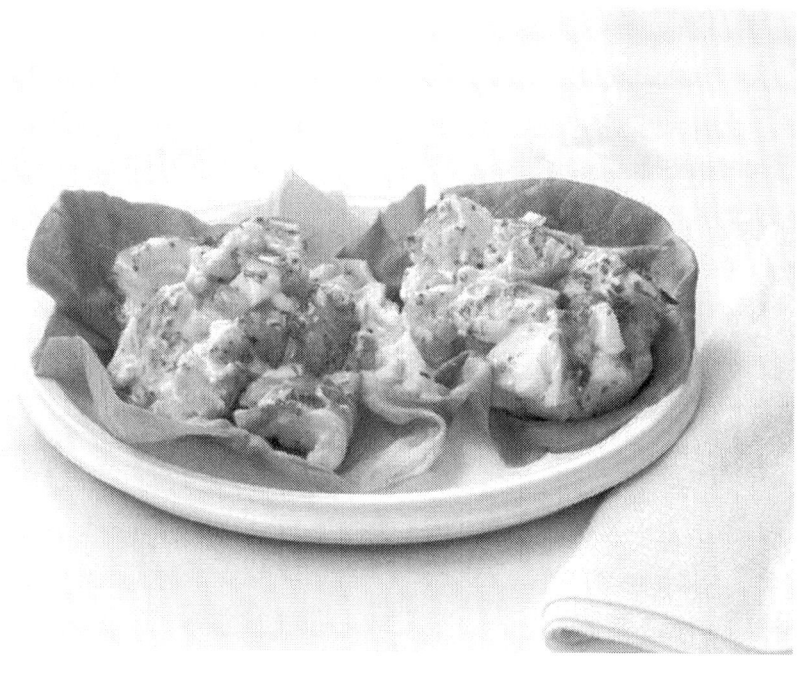

Tandoori Salmon

This recipe makes 2 servings and requires about 15 minutes for cooking.

The serving size is 1/2 salmon. It contains:

- *381 Calories*
- *22 g fat*
- *3 g total, 1 g net carbohydrates*
- *2 g fiber*
- *45 g protein*

What's in It

1 lb	Salmon
2 tsp	Paprika
1 tsp	Garlic powder
1 tsp	Cilantro, dried
1 tsp	Chili powder
½ tsp	Salt
½ tsp	Garam marsala
½ tsp	Turmeric
¼ tsp	Ginger powder
¼ tsp	Pepper
3 tsp	Mustard oil

How's it Made

1. Place tin foil on a baking sheet and heat the oven to 425 degrees Fahrenheit.

2. In a small bowl, combine all the spices with the oil.
3. Place the salmon, skin-side down, on the foiled sheet and rub the spice mixture into it.
4. Place the salmon in the oven and bake for about 5 to 10 minutes. Serve over a plate of spinach or greens.

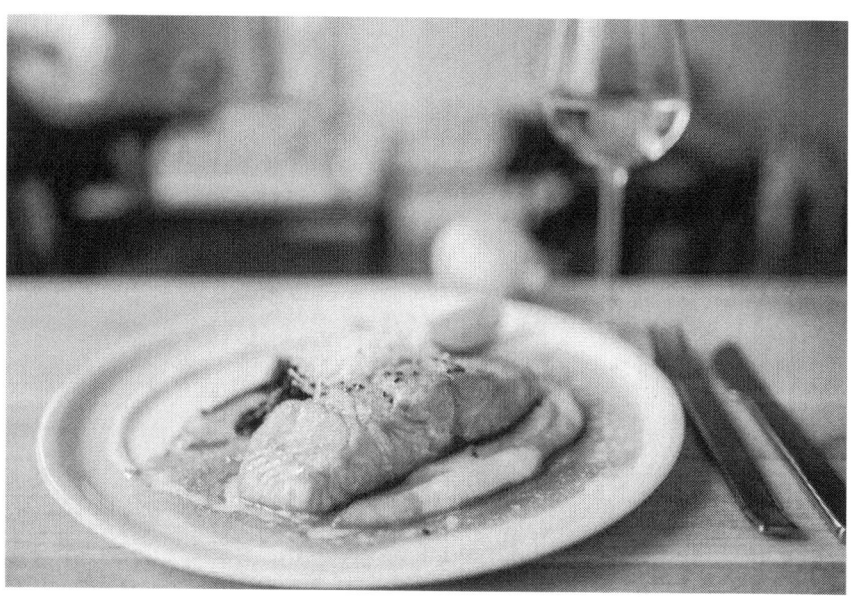

Zucchini "Pasta" and Shrimp

This recipe makes 2 servings and requires about 15 minutes for cooking.

The serving size is 1/2 bowl. It contains:

- *686 Calories*
- *34 g fat*
- *13 g total, 11 g net carbohydrates*
- *2 g fiber*
- *80 g protein*

What's in It

1 C	Shrimp, fresh, cleaned
4 Tbsp	Olive oil
2 cloves	Garlic, minced
1	Lemon, zest and juice
¼ tsp	Salt
To taste	Pepper
2	Zucchini, thinly sliced or spiralized

How's it Made

1. Heat your oven to 400 degrees Fahrenheit.
2. In an ovenproof dish, mix all the ingredients except the zucchini. Place in the oven and bake of about 9 minutes. Remove the dish and stir in the zucchini. Serve warm.

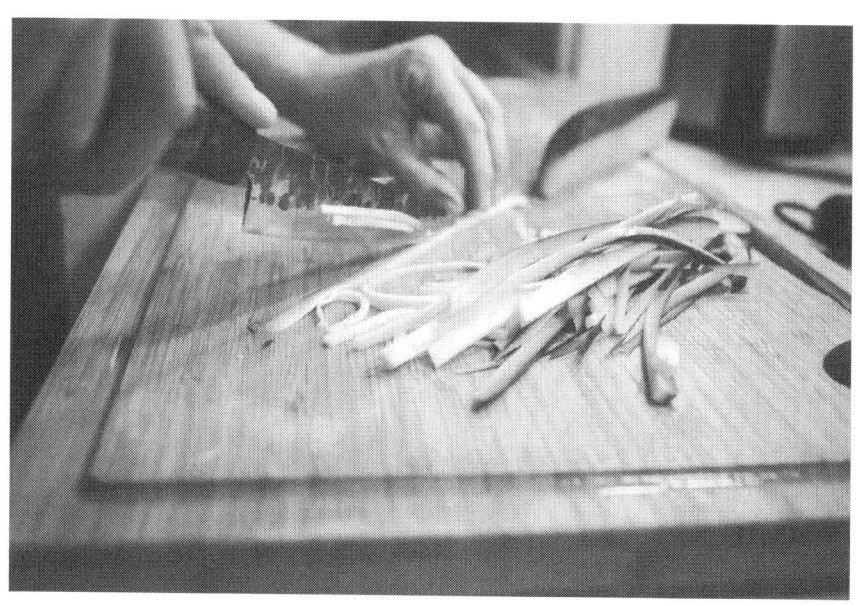

Chicken Fajitas

This recipe makes 4 servings and requires about 10 minutes for cooking.

The serving size is ¼ bowl. It contains:

- *857 Calories*
- *64 g fat*
- *17 g total, 9 g net carbohydrates*
- *8 g fiber*
- *56 g protein*

What's in It

10 Ozs	Lettuce, shredded
5 Ozs	Tomatoes, cherry, halved
2	Avocados, sliced
4 Tbsp	Cilantro, fresh, chopped
3 Ozs	Butter
1 ½ lbs	Chicken, thighs, boneless, sliced
To taste	Salt and pepper
2 Tbsp	Taco seasoning
1	Onion, sliced
1	Bell pepper, sliced
5 Oz	Cheese, jack
1 C	Sour cream

How's it Made

1. In a large skillet, heat the butter over medium-high heat and add the chicken strips.

Sprinkle with salt and pepper as desired. After about 4 minutes, add the peppers, onions, and taco seasoning.
2. Continue stirring and lower the heat to medium-low.
3. In a erring bowl, place the lettuce, cheese, tomatoes, and avocado. Add the chicken mixture on top. Sprinkle with chopped cilantro and the sour cream.

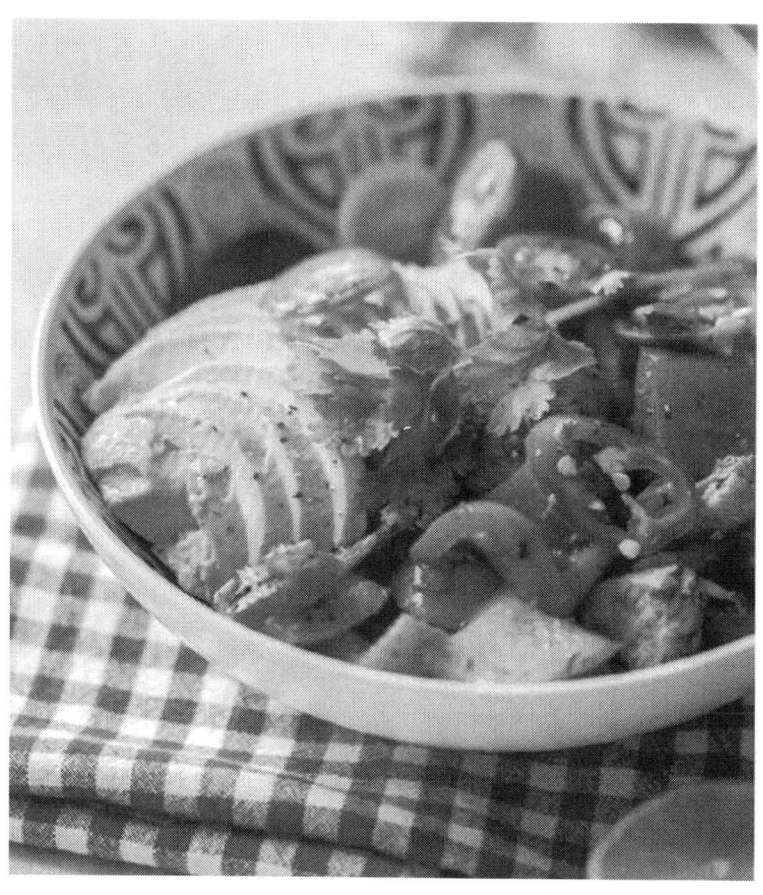

Beef and Brussels Gratin

This recipe makes 4 servings and requires about 15 minutes for cooking.

The serving size is ¼ dish. It contains:

- *902 Calories*
- *63 g fat*
- *36 g total, 26 g net carbohydrates*
- *10 g fiber*
- *50 g protein*

What's in It

1 lb.	Beef, ground
8 Ozs	Bacon, chopped
1 lb	Brussels sprouts, halved
4 Tbsp	Sour cream
2 Ozs	Butter
5 Ozs	Cheese, cheddar, shredded
1 Tbsp	Italian seasoning
To taste	Salt and pepper

How's it Made

1. Heat your oven to 425 degrees Fahrenheit.
2. In a skillet, heat the butter over medium heat and fry the bacon and Brussels sprouts until bacon is crisp. Sprinkle with Italian seasoning and mix in the sour cream.

3. In the same skillet, add the beef, season with salt and pepper as desired, and cook until browned. Add to the Brussels sprouts in the baking dish.
4. Sprinkle the top of the beef and Brussels sprouts with herbs and cheese.
5. Place the baking dish in the oven and cook for 10 minutes or until golden.

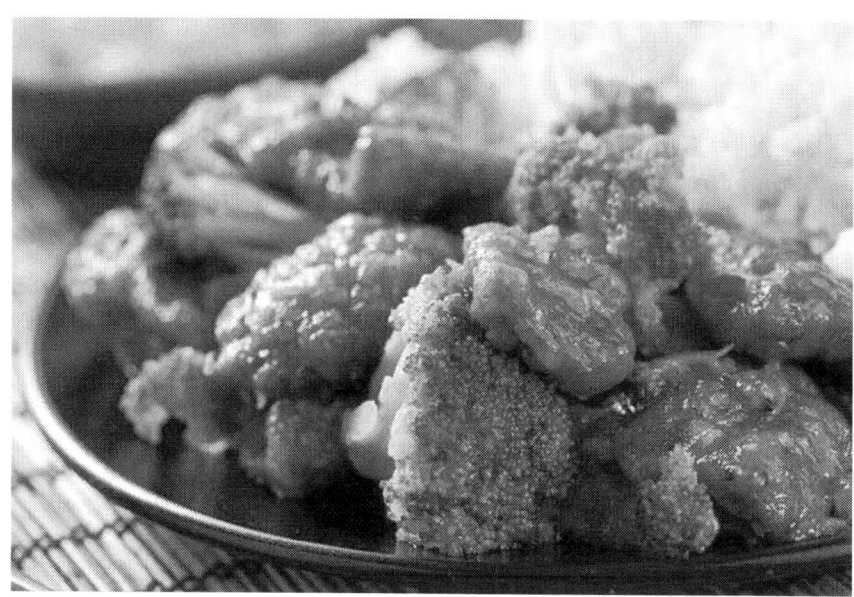

Carbonara

This recipe makes 4 servings and requires about 10 minutes for cooking.

The serving size is ¼ bowl. It contains:

- *860 Calories*
- *80 g fat*
- *9 g total, 7 g net carbohydrates*
- *2 g fiber*
- *25 g protein*

What's in It

1 ¼ C	Heavy cream
2/3 lb	Bacon, chopped
To taste	Salt and pepper
4 Tbsp	Paleo mayonnaise
2 lbs	Zucchini
4	Egg, yolks only
3 Ozs	Parmesan cheese, grated
1 Tbsp	Parsley, fresh, chopped

How's it Made

1. In a saucepan, Boil the heavy cream until only one fourth of it remains.
2. In a skillet, over medium heat, cook the bacon.
3. In the saucepan, stir in the mayonnaise and season with salt and pepper, as desired. Cook until warmed through.

4. Mix the zucchini noodles into the cream sauce.
5. Divide noodles into four servings bowls. Top with bacon, egg, Parmesan, and parsley. Drizzle bacon fat on top, if desired. Serve hot.

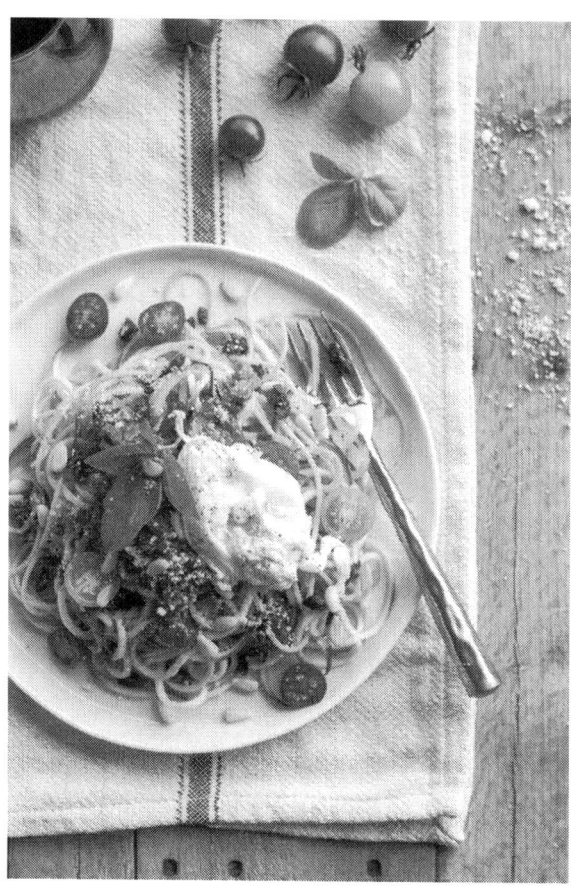

Indian Stir-Fry

This recipe makes 4 servings and requires about 15 minutes for cooking.

The serving size is ¼ bowl. It contains:

- *1038 Calories*
- *97 g fat*
- *9 g total, 4 g net carbohydrates*
- *5 g fiber*
- *31 g protein*

What's in It

1 2/3 lbs	Cabbage, shredded
5 Ozs	Butter
1 lb	Lamb, ground
1 tsp	Salt
1 tsp	Onion powder
¼ tsp	Pepper
1 Tbsp	Vinegar
1 Tbsp	Red curry paste
½	Onion, chopped
8 Tbsp	Cilantro, fresh, chopped
1 C	Paleo mayonnaise

How's it Made

1. In a large skillet, heat ½ of the butter over medium-high heat and fry the cabbage for about 5 minutes.

2. Stir in the vinegar and spices. Sauté for 2 minutes. Put in a bowl.
3. In the same pan, heat the rest of the butter over medium-high heat and combine the curry paste, onion, and garlic. Cook for 1 minute and then add the meat. Cook through and until most of the liquid is gone.
4. Turn the heat down to medium or medium-low and add the cabbage back. Stir well.
5. Top with salt and pepper, chopped cilantro and mayonnaise.

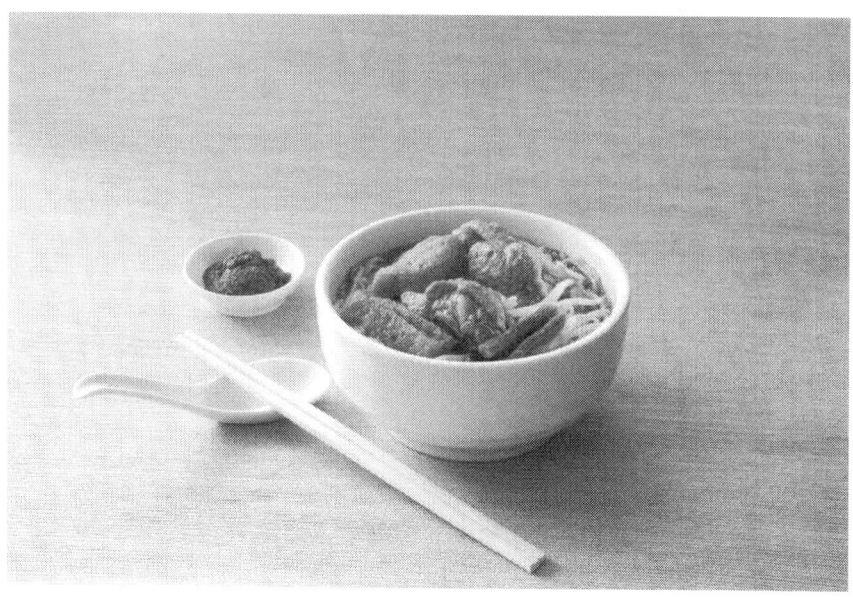

Instant, No-Cook Dinner Options- Grab-and-go

1. Sliced deli meats and pickle spears
2. Fresh spinach, berries and nuts drizzled with olive oil and sprinkled with pepper
3. Salami with sliced avocado and cherry tomatoes
4. Cured salmon with capers, salt and avocado
5. Goat cheese over mixed greens and topped with pecans
6. Smoked salmon mixed with Greek yogurt and fresh, chopped dill served on lettuce leaves
7. Canned tuna served over fresh spinach with cherry tomatoes and olives
8. Prosciutto, fresh mozzarella, sliced tomatoes, and olives served with a mayonnaise or Greek yogurt dip
9. Precooked shrimp tossed in lemon juice and Greek yogurt, served on a bed of mixed greens
10. Roast beef deli meat, cheddar cheese cubes, sliced avocado and cream cheese

Chapter 4
Quick Ketogenic Snacks

Nut and Blackberry Bites

This recipe makes 12 servings and requires about 5 minutes for cooking.

The serving size is 1 bite/ball. It contains:

- *392 Calories*
- *50 g fat*
- *2 g total, 1 g net carbohydrates*
- *1 g fiber*
- *4 g protein*

What's in It

2 ozs	Macadamia nuts, crushed
4 ozs	Cream cheese
1 C	Blackberries
3 Tbsp	Mascarpone cheese
1 C	Coconut oil
1 C	Coconut butter
½ tsp	Vanilla extract
½ tsp	Lemon juice
To taste	Sweetener of choice

How's it Made

1. Preheat your oven to 325 degrees Fahrenheit.

2. In a baking dish, press the nuts into the bottom of the dish and bake for about 5 minutes or until golden. Remove and let cool.
3. Spread cream cheese on the baked nuts.
4. Combine the berries, mascarpone cheese, coconut oil and butter, vanilla, lemon and sweetener and mix until it is smooth.
5. Pour the mixture on the top of the cream cheese and nut "crust" and freeze. This is best after several minutes in the freezer, to allow the topping to solidify.

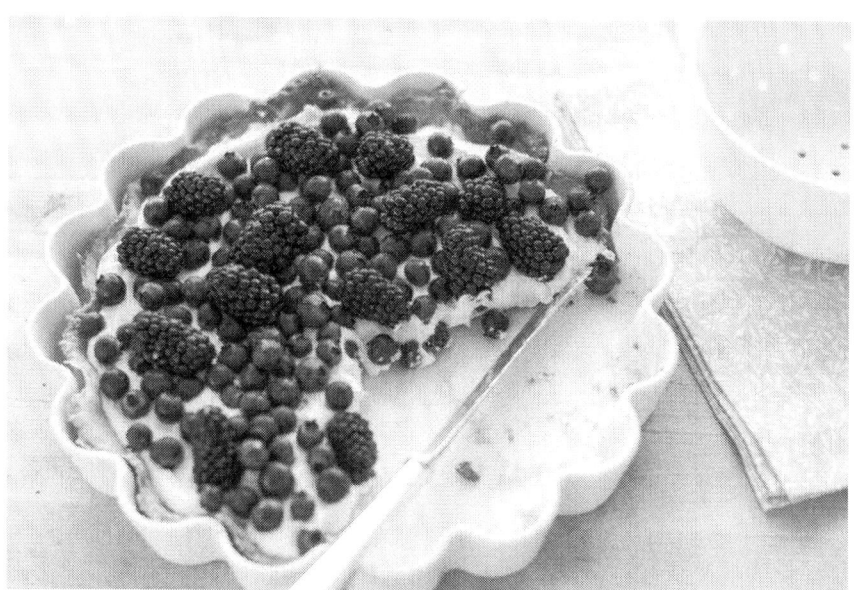

Coconut Bites

This recipe makes 4 servings and requires about 5 minutes for cooking.

The serving size is 3 bites. It contains:

- *644 Calories*
- *65 g fat*
- *17 g total, 7 g net carbohydrates*
- *10 g fiber*
- *5 g protein*

What's in It

1 C	Coconut oil
½ C	Chia seeds
1 tsp	Vanilla extract
1 Tbsp	Honey
¼ C	Coconut flakes, unsweet

How's it Made

1. In a bowl, mix all the ingredients together.
2. Transfer the mixture into muffin tins and place in the freezer until ready to eat. It is best to freeze them for at least 1 hour so the bites have time to solidify.

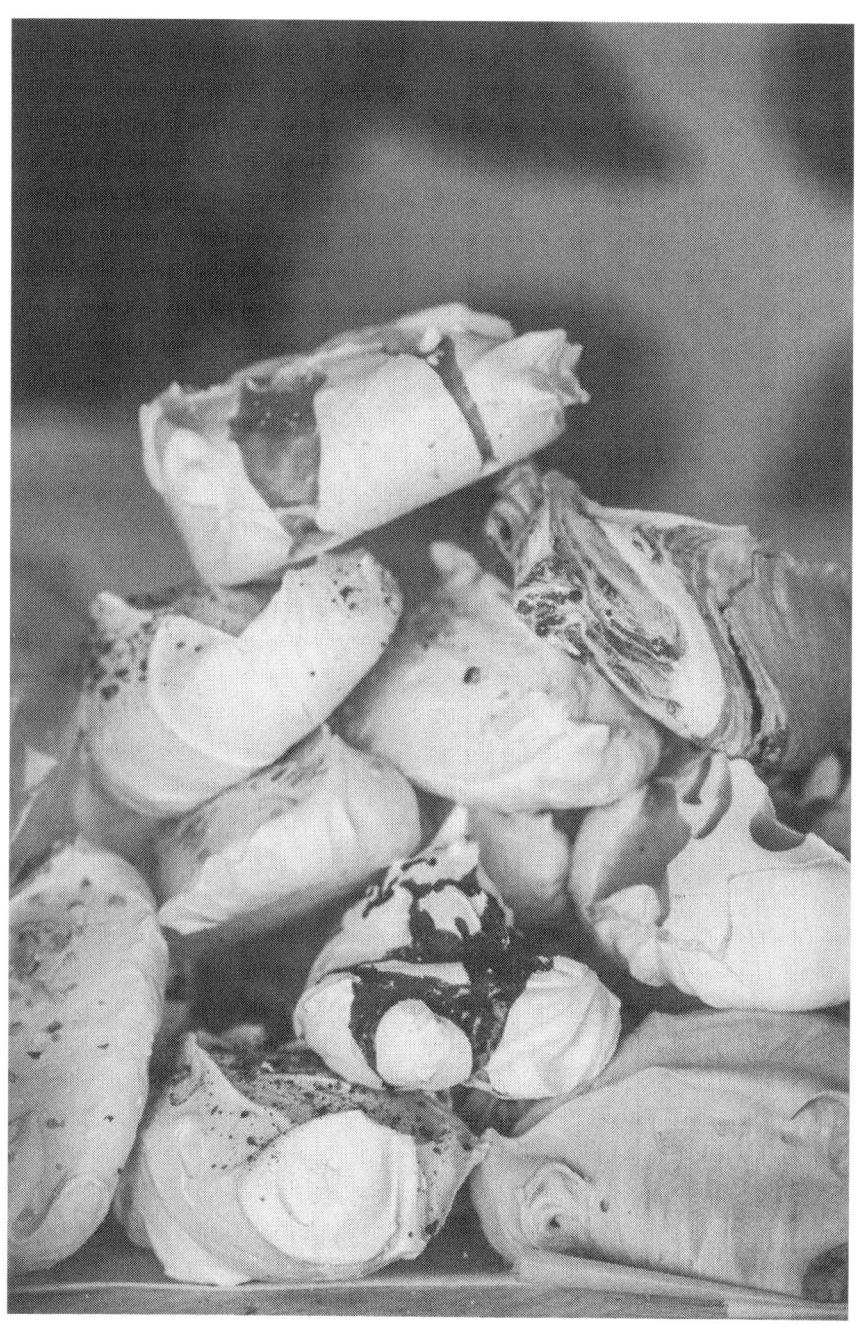

"Tortilla" Chips

This recipe makes 3 servings and requires about 15 minutes for cooking.

The serving size is 10 chips. It contains:

- *157 Calories*
- *11 g fat*
- *2 g total, 1.5 g net carbohydrates*
- *.5 g fiber*
- *12 g protein*

What's in It

½ C	Mozzarella cheese, shredded
¼ C	Almond flour
2 Tbsp	Cream cheese
1	Egg
To taste	Salt
1 tsp	Cumin
1 tsp	Cilantro, dried
Pinch	Chili powder

How's it Made

1. Preheat your oven to 425 degrees Fahrenheit.
2. In a microwave safe bowl, combine the shredded cheese and flour and then mix in the cream cheese. Microwave for 1 minute.
3. Stir the mixture and microwave for another 30 seconds.

4. Stir in the egg, salt and spices.
5. Place the dough between two sheets of parchment and roll out to an even thickness. Remove the top layer of parchment.
6. Place the bottom parchment with the dough on a baking sheet and place in the oven. Bake for about 10 minutes. Turn over onto the top parchment paper, and brown the other side for a few minutes.
7. Remove the tray from the oven, cut into triangular pieces, and bake for 2 more minutes.

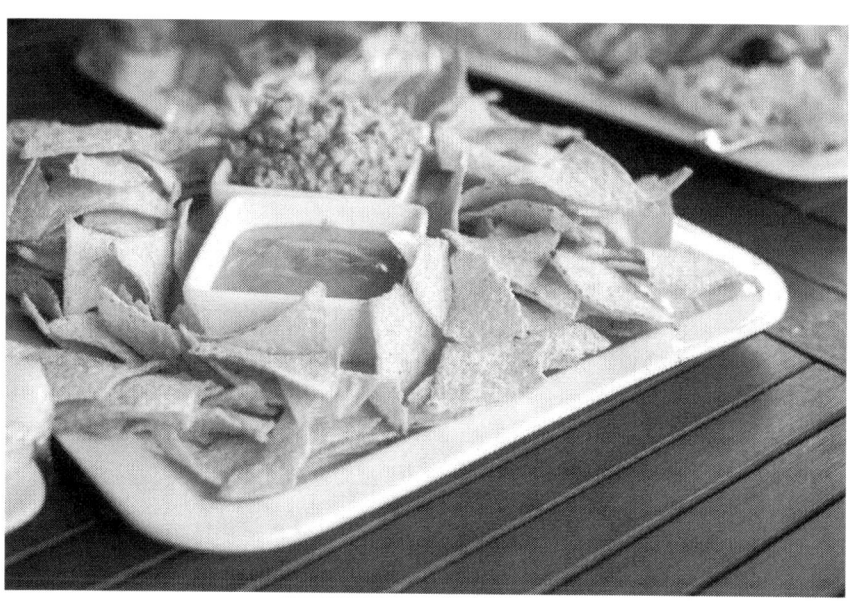

Artichoke Dip

This recipe makes 6 servings and requires about 3 minutes for cooking.

The serving size is 1/3 cup. It contains:

- *475 Calories*
- *36 g fat*
- *10 g total, 6 g net carbohydrates*
- *4 g fiber*
- *31 g protein*

What's in It

1 Can	Artichoke hearts, drained, 14 ozs.
1 lb	Goat cheese
2 Tbsp	Olive oil
2 tsp	Lemon juice
1 clove	Garlic, minced
½ C	Parmesan cheese, grated
1 Tbs	Parsley, fresh, chopped
1 Tbsp	Chives, fresh, chopped
½ Tbsp	Basil, fresh, chopped
½ tsp	Salt
½ tsp	Pepper

How's it Made

1. In a blender or food processor, combine all the ingredients, except for the Parmesan cheese, and mix until a creamy consistency.

2. Spoon into a bowl and top with fresh Parmesan cheese. Eat with fresh sliced vegetables or "tortilla" chips.

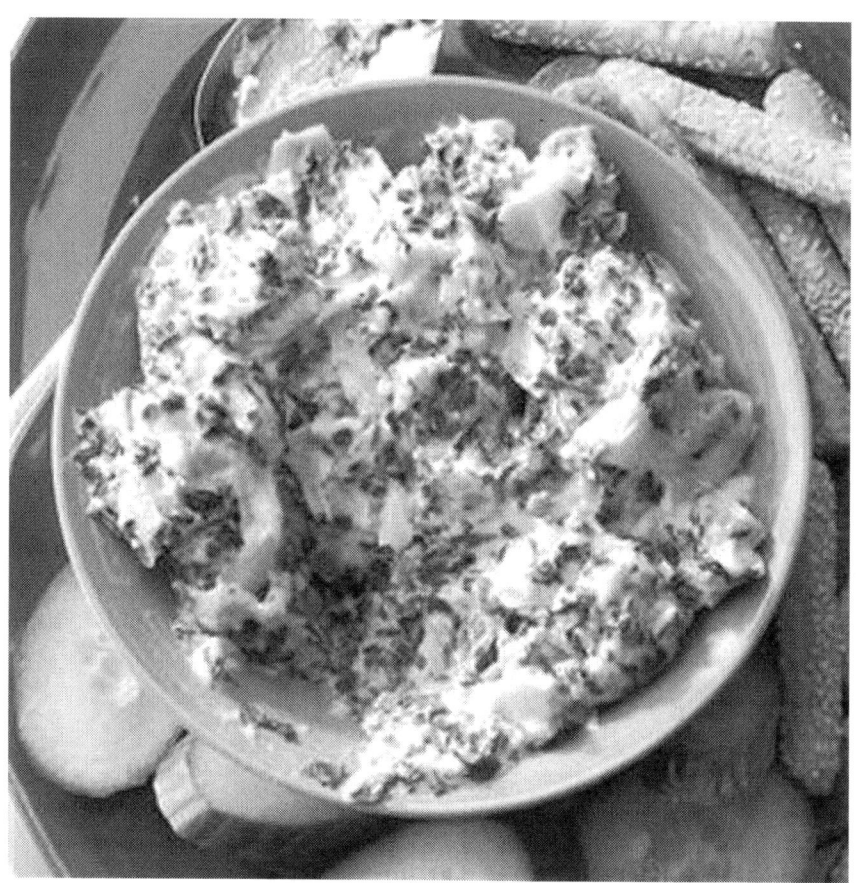

Cheese Crackers

This recipe makes 5 servings and requires about 12 minutes for cooking.

The serving size is 6 crackers. It contains:

- *268 Calories*
- *23 g fat*
- *2 g total, 1 g net carbohydrates*
- *1 g fiber*
- *14 g protein*

What's in It

2 C	Cheddar cheese, shredded
1 C	Almond flour
2 ozs	Cream cheese
1	Egg
½ tsp	Salt
As desired	Garlic, rosemary, dill, chives, etc. for flavor

How's it Made

1. Preheat your oven to 450 degrees Fahrenheit.
2. In a microwavable bowl, combine the cheese and flour and heat for 1 minute.
3. Stir the mixture and allow to cool for a few minutes.

4. Add the remaining ingredients, including flavoring preferences, and stir until well combined.
5. In between two sheets of parchment, place the mixture and roll out until an even thickness. Remove the top layer of parchment and cut the dough into bite-sized squares with a sharp knife or pizza cutter.
6. Place the parchment with the dough onto a try and place it in the oven. Cook for about 5 minutes, then flip onto the original top parchment and place on the tray in the oven to cook for another 5 minutes or until the crisp you desire.
7. Remove from the oven and let cool for a few minutes before eating.

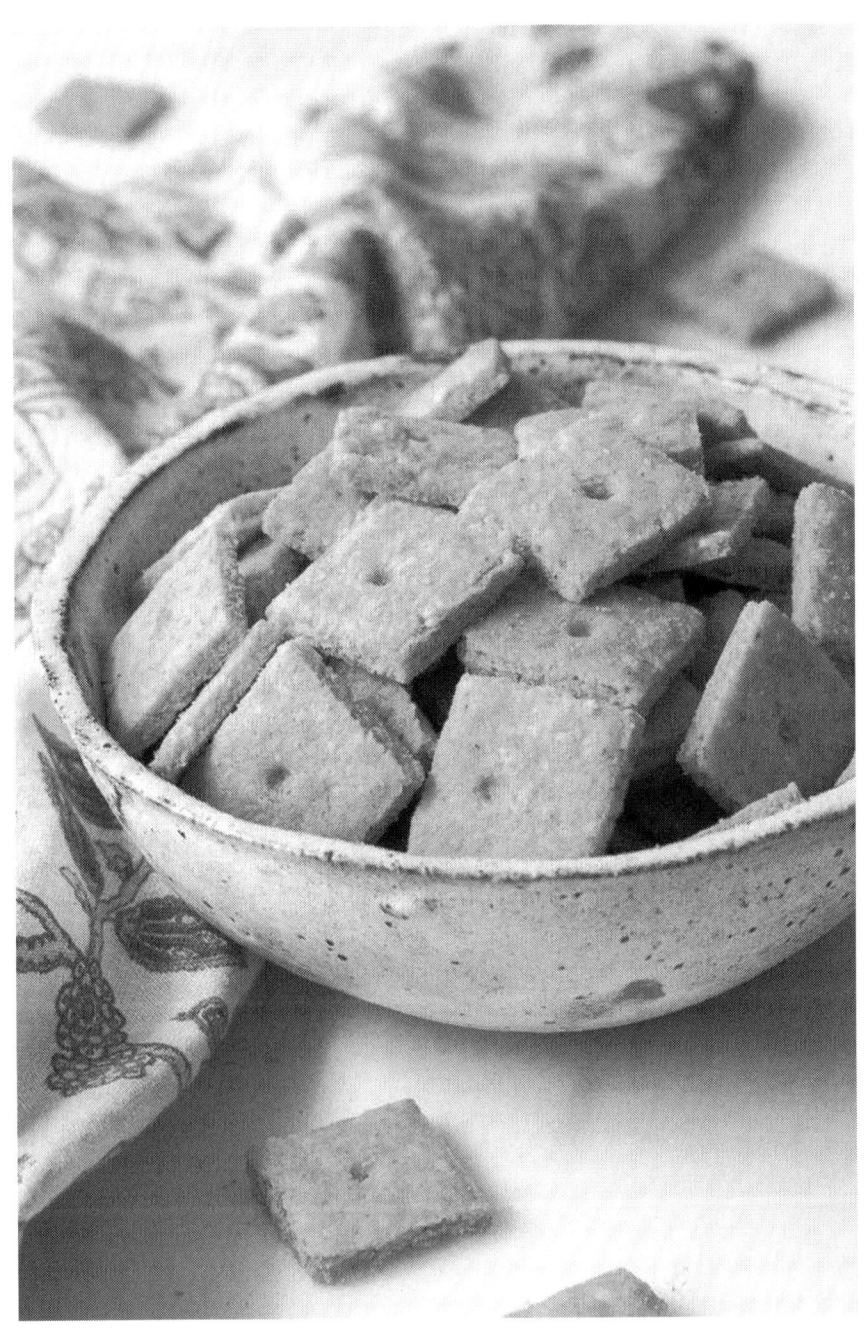

Soft Pretzels

This recipe makes 12 servings and requires about 15 minutes for cooking.

The serving size is 1 pretzel. It contains:

- *217 Calories*
- *18 g fat*
- *3 g total, 1 g net carbohydrates*
- *2 g fiber*
- *11 g protein*

What's in It

3 C	Mozzarella cheese, shredded
4 Tbsp	Cream cheese
1 ½ C	Almond flour
2 tsp	Xanthum gum
2	Eggs, room temperature
2 tsp	Yeast, dry
2 Tbsp	Water, warmed
2 Tbsp	Butter
1 Tbsp	Sea salt or pretzel salt

How's it Made

1. Preheat your oven to 390 degrees Fahrenheit and line a baking sheet with parchment.
2. Place the yeast and warm water in a small bowl and let sit for 2 minutes.

3. In a microwavable bowl, combine the cheeses and heat for 30 seconds, stirring before heating for another 30 seconds. Continue this until all cheeses are melted, typically about 1½ minutes.
4. In a mixer, combine the flour and xanthum gum and mix until combined. Add in the eggs, 1 Tablespoon of butter than has been melted, and the yeast mix. Add the melted cheese slowly and mix for about 3 minutes or until fully combined.
5. Divide the dough into 12 balls and roll into long, snake-like rolls. Twist them into a pretzel shape or another shape you prefer.
6. Place on the lined baking sheet with space between each pretzel. Brush with the remaining tablespoon of butter and sprinkle with salt. Place in the oven and cook for about 11 minutes or until golden. Remove from the oven and allow to cool slightly before serving.

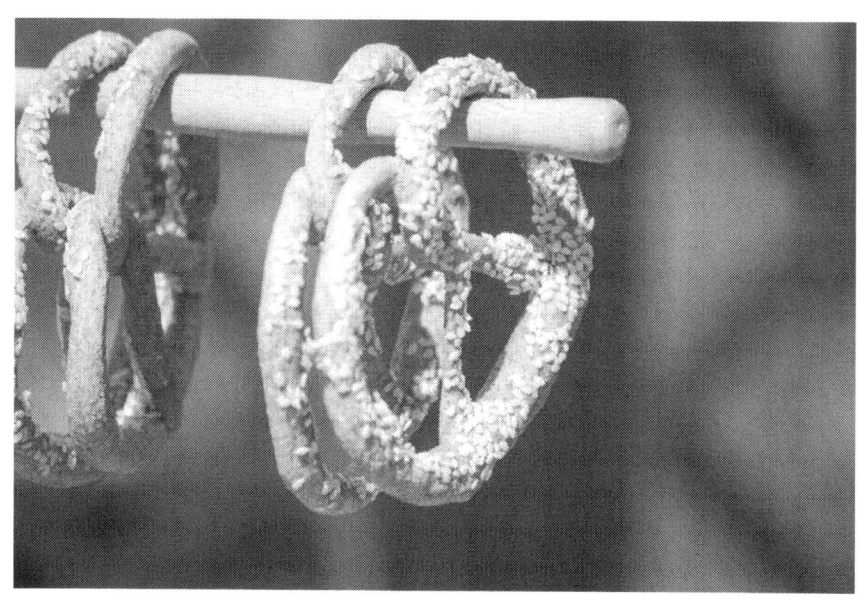

Buffalo "Wings"

This recipe makes 2 servings and requires about 15minutes for cooking.

The serving size is 1½ cups. It contains:

- *175 Calories*
- *11 g fat*
- *10 g total, 3 g net carbohydrates*
- *7 g fiber*
- *4 g protein*

What's in It

3 C	Cauliflower florets
¼ C	Wing sauce
2 Tbsp	Butter
2 cloves	Garlic, minced
Pinch	Salt

How's it Made

1. Heat your oven to 400 degrees Fahrenheit.
2. Brown the butter in a skillet over medium heat. Add the garlic and stir for a few seconds.
3. In a rage bowl, toss the cauliflower with the browned butter and wing sauce.
4. Place the florets, stem side down, in a baking dish and place them in the oven. Bake for about 13 minutes.

5. Remove from the oven and pour the butter and hot sauce mixture on top of the cauliflower. Serve hot.

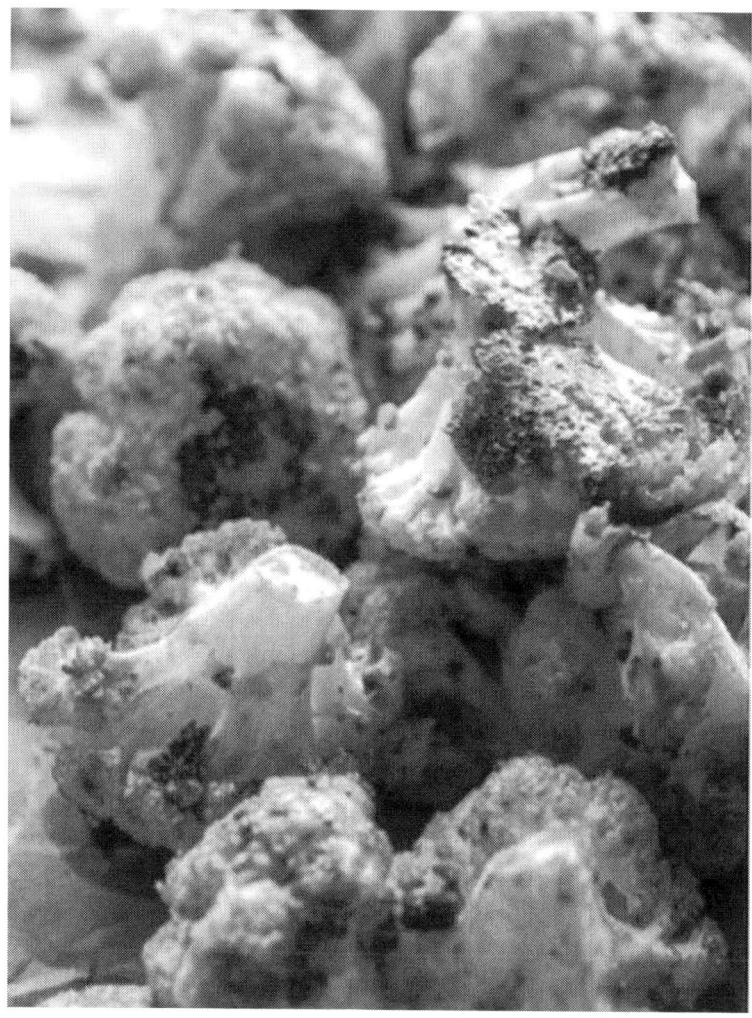

"Ice Cream"

This recipe makes 2 servings and requires about 10 minutes for cooking.

The serving size is 1 cup. It contains:

- *230 Calories*
- *20 g fat*
- *18 g total, 11 g net carbohydrates*
- *7 g fiber*
- *5 g protein*

What's in It

1 C	Cauliflower, steamed, frozen
1 C	Coconut milk, unsweet, full fat
2 Tbsp	Sweetener of preference
10 drops	Stevia, liquid
1 tsp	Pepper
Pinch	Salt
1/3 C	Cocoa powder

How's it Made

1. In a blender or food processor, combine all the ingredients and blend until smooth.
2. Split between two cups and serve immediately.

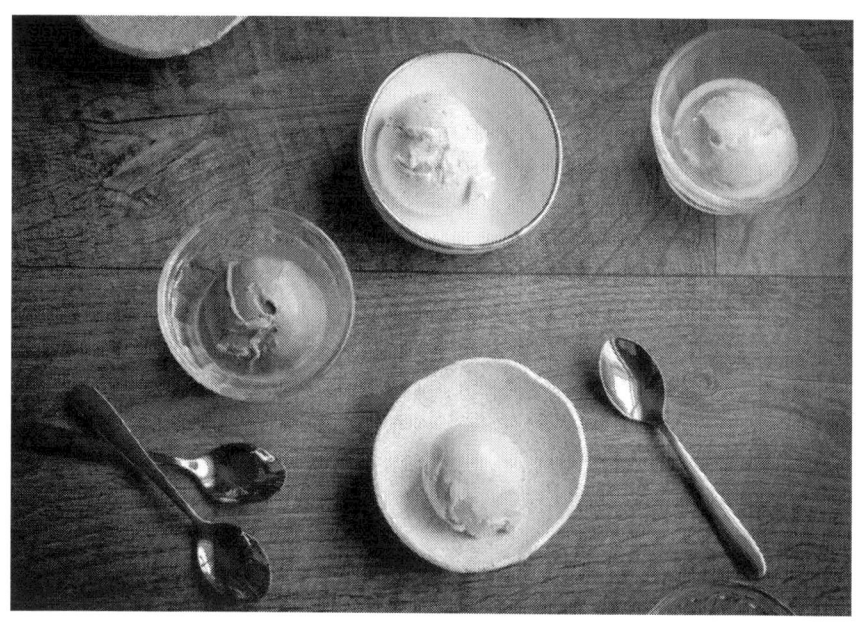

Mint Chocolate Popsicles

This recipe makes 4 servings and requires about 10 minutes for cooking.

The serving size is 1/3 cup. It contains:

- *159 Calories*
- *13 g fat*
- *9 g total, 5 g net carbohydrates*
- *4 g fiber*
- *3 g protein*

What's in It

1 Can	Coconut milk, full fat, room temp
2 C	Mint, fresh
20 drops	Stevia, liquid
1 scoop	Micro greens
Pinch	Cardamom
1 Bar	Dark chocolate bar, chopped

How's it Made

1. In a blender or food processor, combine all the ingredients, except for the chocolate bar, and blend until smooth.
2. In popsicle molds or cups, divide the chopped chocolate evenly and pour in the mint liquid.
3. Place sticks into the molds and freeze until firm.

4. To turn into an instant drink, add ice cubes to the blender and serve with the chopped chocolate.

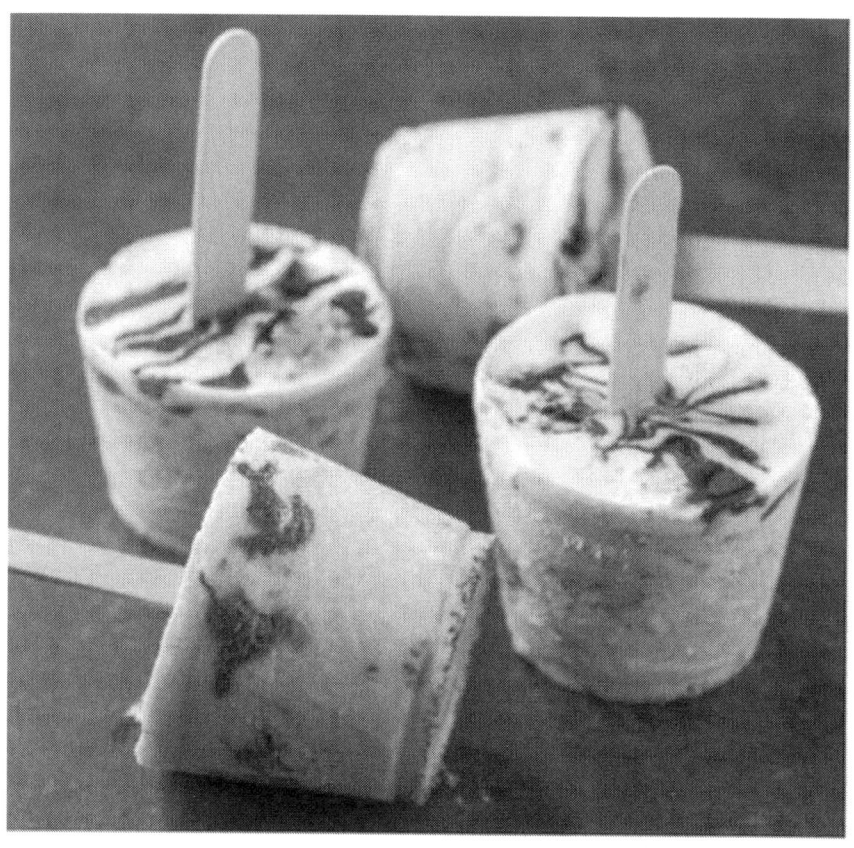

Mousse

This recipe makes 2 servings and requires about 10 minutes for cooking.

The serving size is 1 cup. It contains:

- *188 Calories*
- *14 g fat*
- *13 g total, 6 g net carbohydrates*
- *7 g fiber*
- *3 g protein*

What's in It

¼ C	Blueberries, frozen
½ C	Cauliflower, frozen
½	Avocado
2/3 C	Coconut milk, unsweet, full fat
2 Tbsp	Sweetener preferred
2 Tbsp	Cocoa powder, unsweet
1 tsp	Vanilla extract
1 tsp	Cinnamon
Pinch	salt

How's it Made

1. In a blender, combine all the ingredients and blend until the texture is creamy.

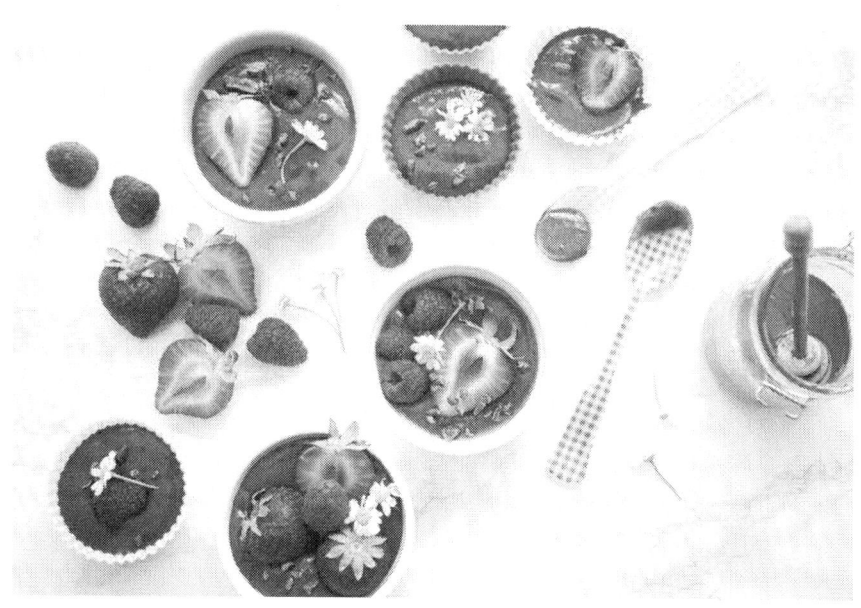

Chocolate Chip Cookie

This recipe makes 20 servings and requires about 15 minutes for cooking.

The serving size is 1 cookie. It contains:

- *191 Calories*
- *18 g fat*
- *12 g total, 2 g net carbohydrates*
- *10 g fiber*
- *4 g protein*

What's in It

1/3 C	Coconut oil, room temp
½ C	Butter
2	Eggs
1 tsp	Vanilla extract
¾ C	Sweetener of choice
½ tsp	Baking soda
¼ tsp	Cream of tartar
½ tsp	Salt
3 C	Almond flour
3 ozs	Baking chocolate

How's it Made

2. Preheat your oven to 350 degrees Fahrenheit and line two baking trays with parchment paper.

3. Mix the coconut oil and butter in a mixer until combined. Mix in the eggs and vanilla extract.
4. Slowly add the sweetener, baking soda, cream of tartar and salt while continuing to mix.
5. Add the flour one cup at a time to the bowl.
6. Heat the chocolate until softened in the microwave while the dough is mixing. Add the chocolate to the mixing bowl.
7. Roll the dough into even-sized balls and place on the trays with space between each ball. Place the trays in the oven and cook for about 12 minutes or until golden.

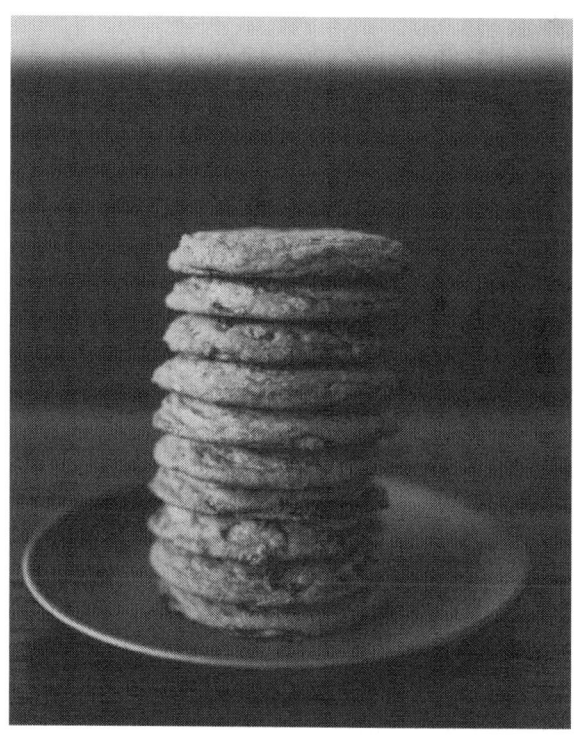

Lemon Cookies

This recipe makes 12 servings and requires about 15 minutes for cooking.

The serving size is 1 cookie. It contains:

- *140 Calories*
- *9 g fat*
- *4 g total, 4 g net carbohydrates*
- *0 g fiber*
- *4 g protein*

What's in It

1 C	Cashew butter
2	Eggs
1	Lemon, zest and juice
½ tsp	Vanilla extract
10 drops	Stevia, liquid
¼ tsp	Baking soda

How's it Made

1. Preheat your oven to 350 degrees Fahrenheit and line two baking trays with parchment paper.
2. Mix the cashew butter, eggs, vanilla, baking soda, and sweetener until combined.
3. Roll the dough into even-sized balls and place on the trays with space between each ball.

Place the trays in the oven and cook for about 12 minutes or until golden.

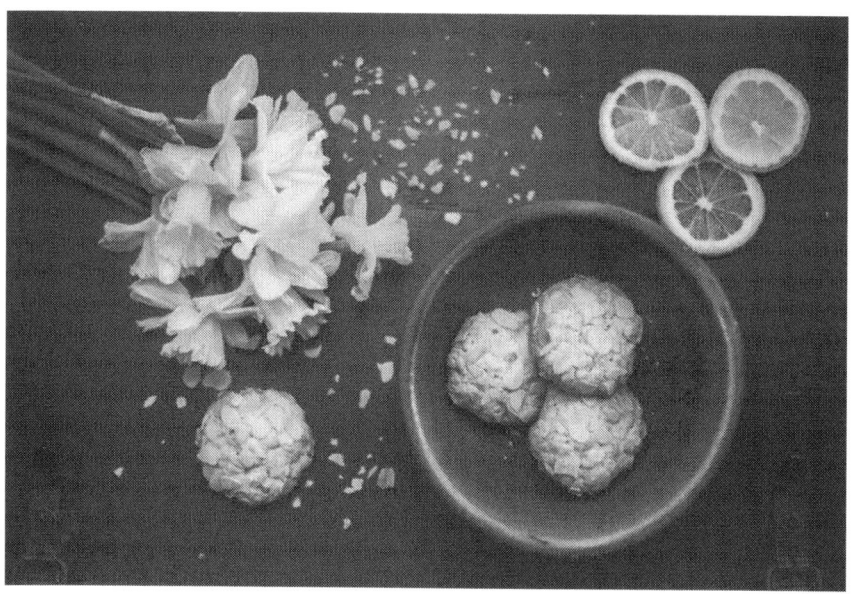

Baked Brie

This recipe makes 4 servings and requires about 10 minutes for cooking.

The serving size is 1/4 cheese round. It contains:

- *345 Calories*
- *31 g fat*
- *3 g total, 1 g net carbohydrates*
- *2 g fiber*
- *15 g protein*

What's in It

9 Ozs	Cheese, brie
2 Ozs	Pecans, chopped
1 clove	Garlic, minced
1 Tbsp	Rosemary, fresh, chopped
1 Tbsp	Olive oil
To taste	Salt and pepper

How's it Made

1. Preheat your oven to 400 degrees Fahrenheit and line a baking tray with parchment paper.
2. In a small bowl, combine all the ingredients except the cheese.
3. Pace the cheese on the tray and top with the herb ad nut mixture. Place the tray in the oven and cook for about 8 minutes or until cheese in softened.

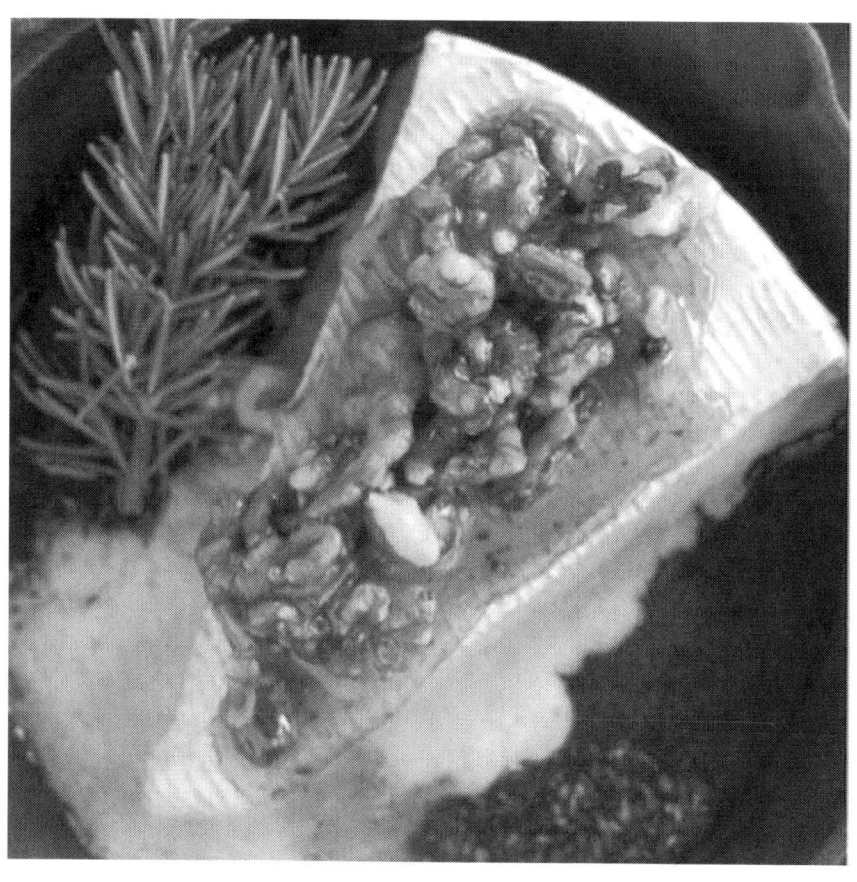

Cardamom Coconut Balls

This recipe makes 10 servings and requires about 5 minutes for cooking.

The serving size is 1 ball. It contains:

- *70 Calories*
- *8 g fat*
- *.5 g total, 0 g net carbohydrates*
- *.5 g fiber*
- *0 g protein*

What's in It

3 Ozs	Butter, room temperature
5 Tbsp	Coconut, shredded, unsweet
Pinch	Cardamom, ground
¼ tsp	Vanilla extract
Pinch	Cinnamon

How's it Made

1. In a small bowl, combine the butter, vanilla, cinnamon, cardamom and ½ the coconut until mixed well.
2. In another small bowl, place the remaining coconut.
3. Separate the dough into 10 even sized balls. Rolls in the remaining coconut. Freeze or cool before serving but can be enjoyed at room temperature.

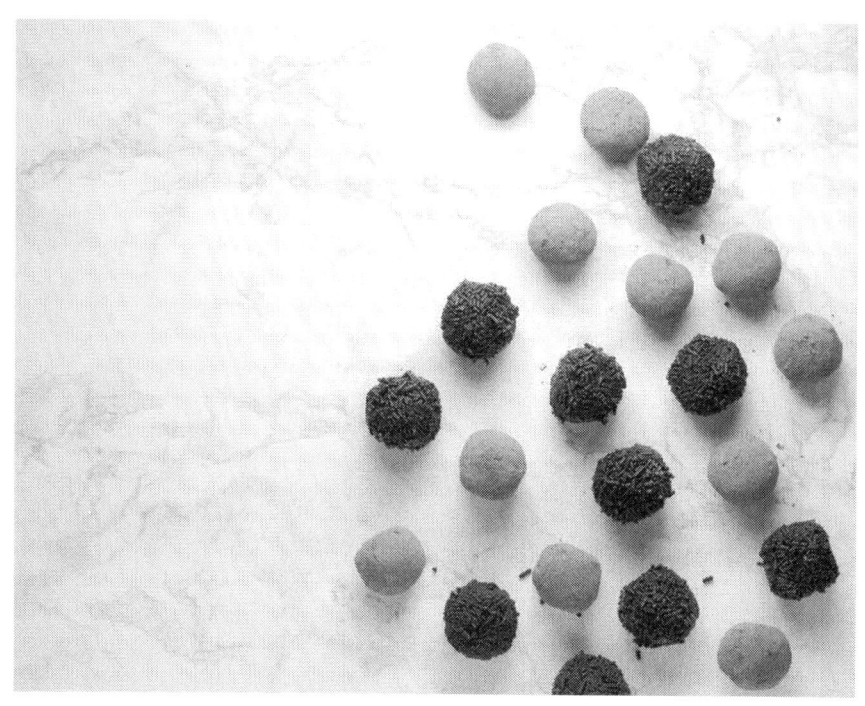

Quick Muffin

This recipe makes 1 serving and requires about 13 minutes for cooking.

The serving size is 1 muffin. It contains:

- *113 Calories*
- *6 g fat*
- *5 g total, 2 g net carbohydrates*
- *3 g fiber*
- *7 g protein*

What's in It

1	Egg
2 tsp	Almond flour
Pinch	Baking soda
Pinch	Salt

How's it Made

1. Preheat your oven to 400 degrees Fahrenheit and oil a small ramekin.
2. In a small bowl, combine the ingredients until smooth. Pour into the ramekin.
3. Place the ramekin in the oven and bake for 12 minutes. Cut in half before serving.

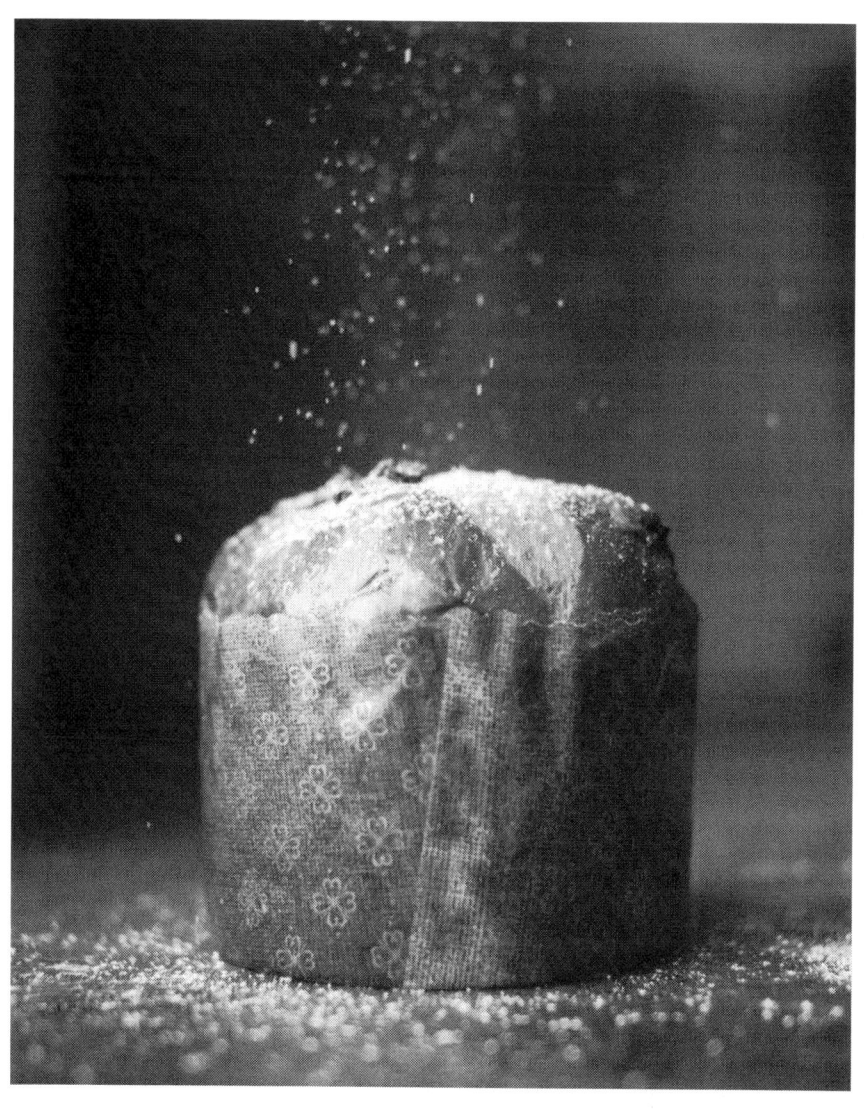

Rosemary and Maple Mixed Nuts

This recipe makes 12 servings and requires about 15 minutes for cooking.

The serving size is 1 cookie. It contains:

- *140 Calories*
- *9 g fat*
- *4 g total, 4 g net carbohydrates*
- *0 g fiber*
- *4 g protein*

What's in It

1 C	Almond
1 C	Pecans
1 C	Walnuts
2 Tbsp	Butter
2 tsp	Maple extract
2 Tbsp	Sweetener of choice
2 Tbsp	Rosemary, fresh, chopped
½ tsp	Salt

How's it Made

1. Preheat your oven to 350 degrees Fahrenheit and line a baking tray with parchment paper.
2. Combine all the nuts in a large bowl.
3. Combine the butter and extract in a small bowl. Add to the nut mixture.

4. Stir in the rosemary and salt and spread onto the baking tray.
5. Place the baking tray in the oven and cook for 10 minutes, tossing frequently.
6. Remove from heat and let cool before serving.

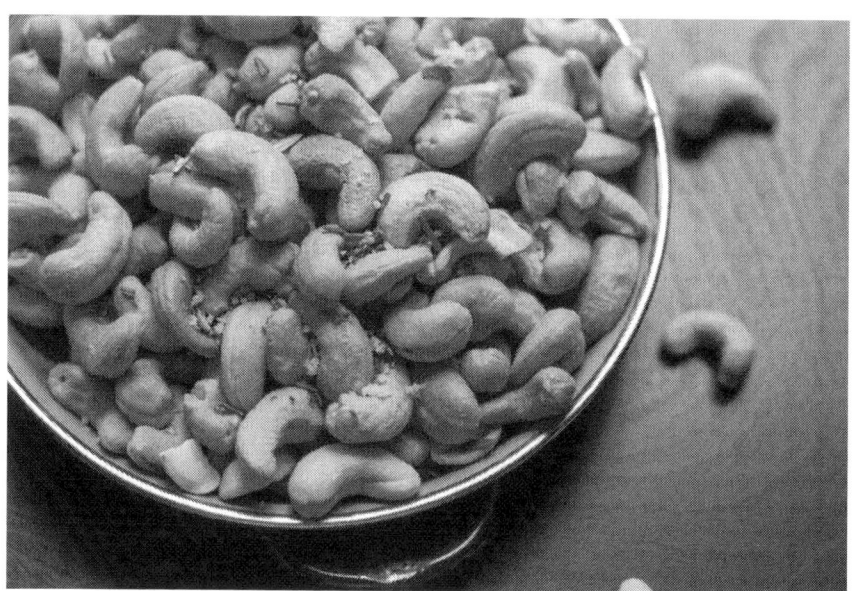

Instant, No-Cook Snack Options- Grab-and-go

1. Avocado slices
2. Deli meat slices
3. Celery sticks with nut butter
4. Handful of nuts and seeds
5. Fresh berries and cheese
6. Variety of cheese cubes
7. Handful of olives
8. Sliced vegetables with mayonnaise or Greek yogurt
9. Cucumber sliced and served with cream cheese and fresh, chopped dill
10. 70% dark chocolate squares
11. Beef jerky

Conclusion

Thank you again for downloading this book, *15-Minute Ketogenic Diet Meals*! I hope it was able to help you feel more confident stepping into your kitchen to create new recipes dedicated to helping you live a healthier and happier life that does not require you to spend hours in the kitchen. You do not have to be a scientist, nutritionist, or doctor to create healthy recipes. You also do not need hours of uninterrupted cooking time to prepare and serve delicious, healthy snacks or meals. You can be a whiz in the kitchen, impressing your friends and family, while serving tasty, fast, and healthy foods. Just tag the recipes in here that you love and everyone will be praising your skills.

The next step in the process is for you to stop reading and drooling over the delicious recipes in this book and go have fun in the kitchen! Remember, you are exploring quick and easy recipes to help you live a healthier life, but you also do not want to deny yourself some of the delicious flavors our global cuisine has to offer. Only you can make the choice to change your diet by making healthier choices. Starting with the variety of recipes in here is one of the ways you can make this ketogenic lifestyle a reality. In your busy life

Finally, if you enjoyed this book, then I'd like to ask you for a favor, would you be kind enough to leave a review for this book on Amazon? It'd be greatly appreciated!

Made in the USA
Lexington, KY
27 June 2018